Beyond the Hippocratic Oath

Beyond the Hippocratic Oath

A memoir on the rise of modern medical ethics

John B. Dossetor

To Kimberly –
with affection
a warm regards

John

The University of Alberta Press

Published by

The University of Alberta Press

Ring House 2

Edmonton, Alberta, Canada T6G 2E1

Copyright © John B. Dossetor 2005

ISBN 0–88864–453–1

Library and Archives Canada Cataloguing in Publication Data

Dossetor, John B. (John Beamish), 1925–

Beyond the Hippocratic Oath : a memoir on the rise of modern
medical ethics / John B. Dossetor.

Includes bibliographical references and index.

ISBN 0–88864–453–1

1. Medical ethics. 2. Nephrologists—Canada—Biography.
3. Physicians—Canada—Biography. I. Title.

RC903.D68 2005   610'.92   C2005–905348–8

Printed and bound in Canada by Marquis Book Printing Inc., Montmagny, Quebec.

First edition, first printing, 2005

The University of Alberta Press is committed to protecting our natural environment.
As part of our efforts, this book is printed on Enviro Paper: it contains 100%
post-consumer recycled fibres and is acid- and chlorine-free.

This book has been subsidized by a Hannah publication grant from the Associated
Medical Services.

The University of Alberta Press gratefully acknowledges the support received for its
publishing program from The Canada Council for the Arts. The University of Alberta
Press also gratefully acknowledges the financial support of the Government of Canada
through the Book Publishing Industry Development Program (BPDIP) and from the
Alberta Foundation for the Arts for our publishing activities.

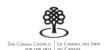

Canada

THE CANADA COUNCIL | LE CONSEIL DES ARTS
FOR THE ARTS | DU CANADA
SINCE 1957 | DEPUIS 1957

Empty is the argument of the philosopher
which does not relieve any human suffering.

—Epicurus, 341 BC–270 BC

Contents

Foreword

CHANGES IN HEALTH CARE IN THE 60 YEARS since World War II have been dramatic, to say the least, and in no area have these changes been more dramatic than in human organ transplantation. Along with the advent of successful treatment for previously fatal illnesses such as chronic kidney disease came the realization that the ethical issues of health care required much more open discussion and public involvement. John Dossetor's medical career has spanned these changes in health care and medical ethics and he has been directly involved in these issues in a very personal way.

Beyond the Hippocratic Oath is a wonderful memoir of an interesting career in medicine that included early training in London, England, experience in India, and a long career in patient care and research at two Canadian academic medical centres: McGill University and the University of Alberta. What comes through clearly in this book is John Dossetor's great personal satisfaction and the intellectual stimulation of being involved in new methods of treatment for patients previously certain to die with chronic kidney disease. Concomitant with these advances in treatment, however, came the ethical challenge of who can receive life-saving treatment among all those who need treatment. Over the years, as research led to greatly improved treatment, the ethical challenges for a thoughtful physician continued to change and multiply, along with the realization that there was much to be learned and taught in medical ethics from a clinician's perspective. The later phase of John Dossetor's career, which also forms the principal theme of this book, involves the remarkable evolution of medical ethics that has accompanied advances in treatment and research. These changes have significantly affected the role of physicians in the doctor-patient relationship—they have taken us "beyond the Hippocratic oath" and now involve all members of an informed public.

The development of life-saving treatment for fatal chronic kidney disease, particularly by kidney transplantation, forms another theme that runs through John Dossetor's book. Before 1960, all patients with end-stage chronic kidney disease died; now many thousands all over the world are alive with kidney transplants or survive on long term artificial kidney (dialysis) treatments. In the past, so little could be done for patients with kidney disease that nephrology did not exist as a distinct area of clinical practice! John Dossetor describes his involvement in the early rudimentary efforts at McGill to remove waste products from the body by intestinal perfusion and the first successful kidney transplantation in the Common-wealth between identical twins. He reveals the medical community's excitement after the dramatic demonstration by Scribner from Seattle that patients with chronic kidney failure could be kept alive for over a year by repeated dialysis treatments; and he describes the first, very limited, success of kidney transplantation from cadaver donors. The advances in clinical and basic research, to which the author and his colleagues at the University of Alberta made important contributions, led to a better ability to match kidney donors and recipients and to more effective ways of controlling the rejection response and, ultimately, to the very high success rates of kidney transplantation today.

At the heart of this book lies the evolution of medical ethics over the past 50 years. This evolution of this field of medicine is as dramatic as the changes that have occurred in the treatment of disease. One of the advantages of a long career in medicine is the opportunity it presents to look back with through the lens of the present day, and John Dossetor takes full advantage of this opportunity. Throughout this book, he inserts personal examples of ethical dilemmas and discusses how, from the perspective of current medical ethics (or bioethics), we would view the events that he describes. These anecdotal experiences taken from his long career in medicine bring to life for the reader the dramatic changes that have occurred in our approach to ethical issues.

From the beginning of life-saving treatment for end-stage kidney disease by dialysis and transplantation, ethical issues have been front and centre: how to select those to receive treatment when available organs or other resources are limited, how to define "brain death" for eligible donors and their families, how to assess quality of life and how to approach possible decisions to discontinue treatment with patients who struggle to survive on dialysis. A triggering event for John Dossetor in his decision to make medical ethics his principal focus was an experience involving a dialysis patient in Edmonton who sought to buy a kidney for himself and later wanted to be allowed to accept a kidney given to him out of "love" from a living unrelated donor. At the same time, there was the realization in the medical school leadership at the University of Alberta that students needed a much stronger educational grounding in medical ethics.

In 1985, John Dossetor therefore embarked on a one-year study leave at several leading centres for health ethics in the U.S. and subsequently returned to launch a new undergraduate teaching program in medical ethics at the Joint-Faculties Bioethics Project (in Medicine and Nursing). The focus of the multidisciplinary team involved in the Project was on issues of clinical ethics that had an immediate relevance for undergraduate students. However, further requests for teaching at the graduate level and in the medical specialties soon emerged. Clinical ethics at the bedside, particularly when faced with life-or-death situations, was evolving from a situation where the doctor's perspective was dominant to a situation where expertise in health ethics and the perspectives of the patient and the family were also very influential. Consequently, Institutional Ethics Committees became common in large hospitals. Examples of difficult moral or ethical decisions at the beginning and end of life are carefully described, together with an effective clinical ethics consultation process. These issues continue as important topics for public discussion today.

The ethics of research in humans, particularly the protection of the rights of patients or volunteers in research, provides another important focus for discussion. Clinical and biomedical research involving humans has grown exponentially since World War II. Physicians who conduct such research are in the position of potentially serving two masters—the patient under their care and the agency funding the research, which may be in the public (government) or private sector. There are many unfortunate past examples of unethical research, but as John Dossetor emphasizes, the rights of the individual patient must always take precedence over the desire to obtain generalizable knowledge through research. He played a key role in the development of national guidelines for research in humans and the establishment of effective institutional research ethics boards that have gone a long way towards creating a sound process for the review and monitoring of such research in Canada.

To return to an area of health or bioethics that first engaged John Dossetor as a young physician, he provides an up-to-date review of the ethical issues associated with human organ transplantation. These issues are numerous and complex, but are fundamentally based on interpersonal relationships, limitations of personal autonomy and what he refers to as "moral intuition." In his concluding chapter, John Dossetor examines the evolution of our approaches to ethical issues through a wide lens—he provides an analysis of the changes in our individual and societal values and the evolution of our ethical ideas or memes and also provides an insightful look into the future.

Beyond the Hippocratic Oath depicts a fascinating period in the history of medicine and highlights the dramatic changes that have occurred in medical care and research in the last 50 years. These events, as well as the even greater changes in health ethics that accompanied them, are told from the personal perspective of a physician who has been directly involved in these very significant changes.

Douglas R. Wilson, M.D., FRCPC
Professor Emeritus of Public Health Sciences and Medicine
Faculty of Medicine and Dentistry, University of Alberta

Acknowledgements

I MUST NOTE THAT THE PEOPLE I have been involved with are the most important influences on my life. Every time I was caught in the car headlights, there was a special person or group of people who triggered the direction of the next jump. They are Ronald Christie, Graham Hayward, Bill Summerskill, Dame Sheila Sherlock, Margaret Conlan (we were married in 1957), John Beck, Moira Johnson, Larry Wesson, Ken MacKinnon, Doug Ackman, Yosh Taguchi, Maisie Strickland, Malcolm Brown, Frank Dixon, Donald Wilson, Walter MacKenzie, Bob Fraser, Calvin Stiller, Ike Bryldt, Ellen Picard, Dorothy Acton, Glenn Griener, Al Jonsen, Vangie Bergum, Doug Wilson, Lorne Tyrrell and Janet Storch. All were critically important at various points in my career. The list of those upon whom I came to depend *after* making these turns would be much longer—too long for this text. But there are several patients' names in the foregoing list who unwittingly played crucial roles. It would be completely false not to acknowledge that the most constant effect on a medical career is the collective support of patients, the people who allowed me the privilege of being involved in their health care decisions. Their gratitude is my reward.

The University of Alberta Press would like to thank Associated Medical Services (AMS) for a Hannah publication grant to subsidize this book. Associated Medical Services Inc. was established in 1936 by Dr. Jason Hannah as a pioneer prepaid not-for-profit health care organization in Ontario. With the advent of Medicare AMS became a charitable organization supporting innovations in academic medicine and health services, specifically the history of medicine and health care, as well as innovations in health professional education and bioethics.

The Press would like also to acknowledge the freelancers who have worked on this book, editor Barbara Sibbald who worked closely with Dr. Dossetor revising and rewriting the manuscript, Halifax freelancer Leanne Ridgeway for fact checking, Peter Midgley for copyediting, Carol Dragich for design and layout, and Wendy Johnson for redrawing the maps in Chapter 7.

Could we then survey the web of thought from the beginning, we should probably perceive it to be at first a chequer of black and white, a patchwork of true and false notions, hardly tinged as yet by the red thread of religion.

But carry your eye farther along the fabric and you will remark that, while the black and white chequer still runs through it, there rests on the middle portion of the web, where religion has entered most deeply into its texture, a dark crimson stain, which shades off insensibly into a lighter tint as the white thread of science is woven more and more into the tissue.

To a web thus chequered and stained, thus shot with threads of diverse hues, but gradually changing colour the farther it is unrolled, the state of modern thought, with all its divergent aims and conflicting tendencies, may be compared.

Will the great movement which for centuries has been slowly altering the complexion of thought be continued in the near future? Or will a reaction set in which may arrest progress and even undo much that has been done?

To keep up our parable—what will be the colour of the web which the Fates are now weaving on the humming loom of time?…will it be white or red? We cannot tell. A faint glimmering light illumines the backward portion of the web. Clouds and thick darkness hide the other end.

— *The Golden Bough: Farewell to Nemi* (1922)
Sir James George Frazer (1854–1941)

Preface

AS A MEDICAL DOCTOR AND PROFESSOR, I have had the privilege of being intimately involved with some epoch-making aspects of change in internal medicine since World War II. I hope that by sharing my collective experiences, together with reflections on both the evolution of medical science and medical ethics during these years, others will gain insight into how important these changes have been and obtain a glimpse of future challenges.

In hindsight, it may seem that my career path was planned and mapped out ahead of time. Nothing could be further from the truth. At one time, I thought of entitling this book: "It all came about by chance...." Afloat on the mainstream of academic medicine in Canada, you might imagine me as a whitewater rafter, coursing ever onwards in exultant anticipation of arriving at some known ultimate destination. Rather, I see myself as a deer by the side of a highway, jumping off in a new direction as each set of headlights startled me to fresh action.

My early career was typical enough, first as a medical student at Oxford University in the 1940s, then working as a junior physician in various teaching hospitals in London, two years of service as a medical officer in the Royal Army Medical Corps with the Ghurkhas in India, and finally training in a London unit for advanced liver disease with a world-famous group. A sudden decision to move to the Royal Victoria Hospital, part of McGill University in Montreal in 1955, my emigration to the U.S. in 1960, and my to return to Montreal a year or so later changed my direction entirely. Once resettled in Canada, a pattern seemed to emerge in the specialty of fluid, electrolytes, and acid-base pathophysiology, leading to specializing in kidney diseases—destined to be called nephrology. Then, again, random chance precipitated me into kidney transplantation in 1963, after a foretaste of its potential in 1958. Research in this area led to a move to the University of Alberta Hospital in Edmonton in 1969. All this was subsumed, in its turn, by an increasing commitment to health ethics, and in 1985 I accepted a full-time appointment in health ethics at the University of Alberta. None of these personal evolutions were planned.

I can perceive how my career choices are integrated into two wider themes: rapid medical advances and the burgeoning importance of bioethics, or health ethics. My personal and professional experiences, especially in the fields of kidney disease, medical and health ethics, and the emerging field of applied human values in health care, are all intertwined in this memoir. Looking back, I am able to discern, in the blend of past events, dominant themes that were not really apparent at the time.

The changes in health care and the management of human afflictions during the last 50 to 60 years have been enormous. I start my retrospective journey here by tracing the evolution of medical knowledge in its different disciplines, identifying key factors and epoch-making events that would, unbeknownst to me, shape my medical career. Since World War II there has been an explosion in understanding of the mechanisms of disease, the means of investigating how a disease process causes its effect, determining what precisely is functionally deranged and, most important, the steps that can be taken to restore health. This explosion was encouraged and supported by an enormous increase in funding for basic and clinical research and the incredible growth of the pharmaceuticals industry and associated technologies, both diagnostic and therapeutic. My career, and that of my colleagues, benefited immensely from this new infusion of interest in research.

From this evolution of medical knowledge came a concurrent evolution of medical or health ethics. The topic of health care ethics never surfaced in the curriculum of a medical student trained 60 years ago. Instead, there was a tacit understanding that the art of medicine began and ended with the way in which one treated patients as individuals within the sanctuary of the doctor-patient relationship, though what this relationship was not discussed—it was more or less assumed.

Underlying this relationship was the Hippocratic tradition and its fundamental tenet of bringing benefit to the patient and above all doing no harm. But this was steeped in professional paternalism, the idea that "doctor knows best." Notions of consent, except for clear-cut events such as surgery, were still quite rudimentary. The concept of the patient as a joint or participatory informed decision-maker making comprehended choices among alternatives simply did not exist. The phrase "promoting patient autonomy" would have been considered pure hyperbole. But now, health ethics plays a central role in all aspects of medical and health care and research. How and why has this vast change occurred? What were the seminal steps in that progression?

As a participant in both of these evolutionary trends, I hope my personal experiences can contribute to answering these questions. In the field of health ethics, it is easy now to see previous shortcomings, both personal and collective. In that sense many experiences recounted in this book may seem to be as much an *apologia* as they are a dispassionate account of an evolutionary process.

At an individual level, everyone, whether or not he or she acknowledges it, is an ethicist—and an experienced one, at that. We all make ethically significant decisions every day of our lives. We all consider what is right and wrong based on what we perceive to be good or bad. We all believe we *ought* (an ethically loaded word) to do this or that, and no other person has greater insight into our world of decisions, or indeed responsibility for the decisions we make, than we do. These obligations and responsibilities are part of the process of being an adult and having relationships with others—family, neighbours, patients, friends and colleagues—with whom we share our values.

Although it is true that some make a special study of certain ethics issues or become familiar with the aspects of certain issues because of repeated exposure, the fact remains that all of us have views on the ethical problems we face and are the prime authority for making these ethical decisions. We can be as sure about the ethical probity of our own carefully deliberated opinions on an issue as that of a so-called expert ethicist, especially on everyday or "small-ticket" decisions, such as respect for people. For these reasons, ethics is different from the law, medical science, or mathematics.

But there are also ethical decisions to be made within the context of these specialties. Medical science, which often involves life and death or quality of life, "big-ticket" decisions, demands a more technically informed and considered approach. Rational thought and consideration outside the emotional confines of illness, accident and its attendant distress, and beyond the pecuniary interests of some research funding groups, is essential to ethical decision-making at this level. Although by necessity these decisions are often fraught with technical and scientific detail, often they can be distilled into fundamental ethical questions that can be intuitively grasped by a lay person. With this understanding comes a move away from the paternalistic pattern of medicine toward a more consensual and informed approach.

My hope is that this book helps the reader understand why this move is necessary in the context of modern medicine, how it evolved and now functions, and the challenges we now face. As I quoted at the start of this preface: "A faint glimmering light illumines the backward portion of the web."

I. Early Days

I swear by Apollo Physician and Aesculapius etc....I will apply dietetic measures for the benefit of the sick according to my ability and judgment; I will keep them from harm and injustice.

I will neither give a deadly drug to anybody who asked for it nor will I make a suggestion to this effect. Similarly I will not give to a woman an abortive remedy. In purity and holiness I will guard my life and my art.

I will not use the knife, not even on sufferers from stone, but will withdraw in favor of such men as are engaged in this work.

Whatever houses I may visit, I will come for the benefit of the sick, remaining free of all intentional injustice, of all mischief and in particular of sexual relations with both female and male persons, be they free or slaves.

What I may see or hear in the course of the treatment or even outside of the treatment in regard to the life of men, which on no account one must spread abroad, I will keep to myself, holding such things shameful to be spoken about.

If I fulfil this oath and do not violate it, may it be granted to me to enjoy life and art, being honored with fame among all men for all time to come; if I transgress it and swear falsely, may the opposite of all this be my lot.

— *Hippocrates (460 BC to c. 370 BC)*[1]

Witnessing the dawn of a new epoch:
The advent of a wonder drug

WE CALLED HER PROF. BULBRING. Her husband probably called her Eva, or some more particular endearment. She taught pharmacology to medical students during World War II at Oxford University Medical School. I was there in her class, along with 70 others, in 1943 at the age of 18, despite being old enough to be drafted for military service. The assumption was that we would soon be medical officers. How well did she teach? I cannot really remember, so I think it can be assumed that she taught well enough, but not outstandingly so. She was not as flamboyant and startling as Dr. Alice Carleton, who, with grey hair dyed a steely blue, drew multicoloured anatomical illustrations on the board in her very well-attended anatomy lectures on the peritoneal membrane or the human genitalia. Nor did Prof. Bulbring have the *gravitas* of Prof. Le Gros Clarke, the professor of anatomy who had described a very ancient prehistoric skull during his anthropological scientific past (though this finding was subsequently discredited). Prof. Bulbring was not famous in that sense, but she was destined for fame.

One day, Prof. Bulbring sustained a compound fracture of her ankle in a bicycle accident. The skin was broken and the joint exposed. It was a serious accident with a high risk of joint infection and subsequent osteomyelitis, a condition where the dead bone causes an inflammatory infection in the adjacent bone. In those days, the normal treatment was to amputate the foot. Not that an infected joint could not suppurate properly and effectively drain itself, or be drained of its pus, but the effect of such a process would be joint fusion and continued infection, after which the foot would be relatively useless. One would be better off with an artificial foot and a well-healed stump. It could be assumed that such was the fate in store for Prof. Bulbring.

But in Oxford at that time a new drug called penicillin had recently been developed for difficult infections, although no one knew much about it. It came from the laboratory research in the William Dunn School of Pathology, part of the medical school complex next door to where we were studying pharmacology. Prof. Bulbring was offered this drug as a way to avoid the disastrous effects of an infected ankle joint and amputation. She accepted. Her joint was repaired and it healed under the protective cover of penicillin injections without residual harm to the joint. She was one of the very first people in the world to receive the drug and this fact, and her obvious recovery, was made known to the medical students and made a lasting impression on all of them, not least myself.

When Prof. Bulbring received her experimental injections, there was no mention of any possible ethical dilemma. In fact, during my four years at St. John Baptist College at Oxford, and subsequent three-and-a-half years of pre-graduation clinical training at St. Bartholomew's Hospital Medical School in London (Bart's, as it is known), there was no mention

Ethical Dilemma

Were the dangers of this experimental therapy explained to Prof. Bulbring? Probably not. Very little was known about possible toxicity except that the two principal researchers had shown that it was non-toxic to animals. Did she give informed consent? Well, she consented no doubt, and she certainly knew of alternative treatments, but the amount of information must have been limited. Was she part of a controlled trial? No, she definitely was not. For the surgeons at that time, she might have been part of a pilot study or even part of what, in today's parlance, would be called a Phase I trial. But in reality, she was treated under the rubric of "innovative therapy" leading possibly to a pilot study. However, her exposure to penicillin was justified by the immediacy of the need and the available evidence of non-toxicity in animals. And there was enough experience— from data usually referred to as historical controls—to know that amputation was otherwise indicated. It was fortunate, indeed, that penicillin did not have delayed kidney or liver toxicity when given to humans.

of the possible significance of ethics in medicine. In retrospect, however, this case did present ethical dilemmas.

What this event illustrated was that contemporary human research ethics was not yet born. The only country that had an articulated system of human research ethics during this era was pre-World War II Germany, which was tragically destined to ignore it from 1936–1947.[2] (Details on the German research ethics code are given in Chapter 12.)

PENICILLIN: THE EMERGENCE OF A WONDER DRUG

In 1922, Alexander Fleming (1889–1955), a bacteriologist at St. Mary's hospital in London, first detected an antibacterial enzyme—lysosyme—in nasal mucus. He noted this after a sneeze over an open culture plate inhibited the growth of bacteria. In 1928, he discovered through another chance happening—accidental exposure of a culture plate to air—a mould that inhibited culture plate growth, and called this mould *Penicillium notatum*. He realized it had unusual bactericidal properties against staphylococci, and used it to clean up his culture plates in the laboratory. For him it was a bacterial weed killer, nothing more, though he noted that it only worked against some strains of bacteria. He did not think of any possible application to infection in humans or, indeed, in any animal tissues.

About eight years later, Howard Florey (1898–1968) and biochemist Ernst Chain (1906–1979)—the latter a refugee from the Jewish pogroms in Nazi-dominated Europe—were trying out a number of compounds for control of infection in humans. They took the reports of Fleming's "bacterial weedkiller" mould and explored it for its safety in controlling infections in animals or humans. They quickly realized that penicillin extract cured certain infections and appeared to be well tolerated without any obvious toxicity.

Penicillin was first used on a human with a severe infection at an Oxford hospital. Albert Alexander, a policeman, improved dramatically only to relapse and succumb when they ran out of penicillin. In 1941, Florey and his team began growing large amounts of the mould at Oxford, but ended up going to the U.S. for help in making enough to begin clinical trials. By 1941, the U.S. government and private industry began commercial production of penicillin. Fleming, Florey and Chain shared the Nobel Prize in Physiology and Medicine in 1945. For the most balanced account of these events, see Eric Lax, *The Mold on Dr. Florey's Coat*, New York: Henry Holt, 2004.

Penicillin was soon heralded as a panacea against infections, especially those caused by meningococci, pneumococci, staphylococci, streptococci, gonococci and the dreaded *Typanosoma pallidum* of syphilis. At that time, pneumococcal pneumonia—or lobar pneumonia—carried a 20 per cent mortality. A year or so after penicillin became available, this rate fell to less than five per cent.[*3] Penicillin heralded the revelations of medical science that flowered in the post-World War II epoch. It showed how dramatically infections could be controlled, although little attention was paid to the possibility of harm.

Later, I realized that this was my first brush with medical ethics—an area that would become a cornerstone of my career as it dovetailed medicine's unprecedented advances over the next 60 years. These advances brought to the fore the need for a more formal understanding and use of medical ethics to make appropriate decisions.

To fully appreciate these advances, consider the changes that have occurred in health care over the last 240 years or so using the relatively simple criterion of length of life, or longevity (see Figure 1.1). I have divided modern medical history into four epochs: circa 1760 to 1880; 1880 until the start of World War II; 1940 to 2000; and, the fourth epoch, the start of the new millennium until 2060, which is of necessity largely speculative (see also Appendix 1). This figure is conjectural; the data are culled from various estimates and illustrate a general idea of the evolution of medical care for those in the industrialized West—the affluent 20 per cent or less of the world's population. Note how the percentage of those who survive to 65 has increased in the present epoch from 40 to 64 per cent.

This increase in longevity corresponds with changes in knowledge of disease. The **first epoch** (circa 1760–1880) precedes the time when micro-organisms (bacteria, fungi, viruses and the like) were known to cause infectious disease. The medical armamentarium included such "remedies" as digitalis (William Withering, 1775), lime juice for scurvy, quinine, morphine, tartar emetic, bromides, enemas, as well as clysters, cupping, nostrums and blood letting. Many infants and children did not survive, and only 25 per cent of people reached old age. Surgery was commonly

---

* Looking back, we know that the case fatality rate for pneumococcal pneumonia was 30 to 35 per cent among adults in the 1930s and that it fell to 20 to 25 per cent with the advent of serum containing anticapsular antibody, to 12 to 15 per cent with the availability of sulfonamides, and eventually to 5 to 8 per cent with the introduction of penicillin. Wenzel RP, Edmond MB. Managing antibiotic resistance [editorial]. *N Engl J Med* 2001;343(26):1961–3.

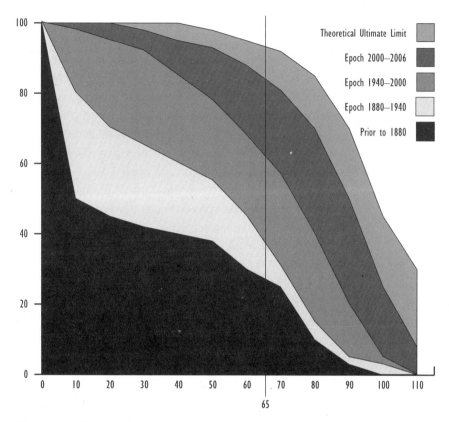

Figure 1.1 Increasing longevity in the Western world.

This longevity curve shows the percentage of the population surviving through each decade for four successive epochs of Western health care. (Note: Infant mortality rates for the period 1760–1880 are not plotted here because the curves only refer to those who survived the first month or so of life.) See Appendix 1 for further details about the four epochs.

practiced on injured limbs and amputations were often successful. However, those wounded in war were much more likely to die of infection than of the injury itself, and surgery within the abdomen, thorax or skull was extremely hazardous and seldom undertaken.

Health and longevity improved during the **second epoch** (1880–1940) largely due to a growing understanding of the bacterial causation of disease and antisepsis (infection); the importance of clean water, good drains and sewers; and the protection that came from the early science of immunizations and vaccination. Still, apart from insulin (1923) and thyroid extract, there were few specific therapies for specific diseases. However, during this period, different diseases became increasingly understood and the natural history of each described—even though little could be done to alter their course.

Although this book concentrates on ethical issues that have come to the fore during the last four or five decades (the third epoch), it would be quite false to give the impression that ethical issues had not arisen previously. Consider vaccination for small pox as an example. In 1855 at Boston, all children had to be vaccinated before attending public school. Most children were vaccinated voluntarily on the authority of their parents. But what would this society do in the event of an outbreak? In 1901, that is precisely what happened, and it was believed at the time that unvaccinated homeless people were the cause of the spread. Their answer was to forcibly vaccinate those individuals against their will. This gave rise to great concern and various legal challenges at the state and federal levels. In the end, the issue was decided in favour of the State by the Supreme Court in 1905, on the grounds that the public good outweighed individual rights.[4]

At the beginning of the **third epoch** (1940–2000), when the body was broken, it could be repaired to some extent; where there was pain, one could try surgical or physical methods to assuage that pain within the narrow constraints of anesthesia and surgery, and morphine. Apart from this, there were serious therapeutic limitations. In short, there was much caring—arguably, considerably more than nowadays—but not much that could be called curing.

Since 1940, the knowledge of physiology, pharmacology, anesthesiology and biochemistry and, thus, the mechanisms of diseases, have grown exponentially. Each area of science created the potential for development in another. For example, the transformation of anesthesiology enabled enormous advances in surgery. As well, dramatic advances in biology, evolutionary biology, inorganic and organic chemistry and physics allowed medicine to evolve further. Not surprisingly, medical and surgical specialties have increased from about ten in 1940 to some 40 today.

There has also been an enormous expansion in pharmaceuticals as powerful tools against disease and infection. In 1940 there were fewer than 100 approved drugs; today there are over 1,000. These drugs are more specific and potent than their predecessors, making the need for accurate medical diagnosis much more important. In fact, it becomes more important with every new powerful agent that has the power to do good, because it also has the power to do harm. This need to assess benefit accurately underlies the great upsurge in medical research—in randomized controlled clinical trials, in the emergence of health care legislation, and litigation against professionals when things go wrong—and the emergence of health ethics.

Thus, in 60 years, medicine was transformed from a somewhat impotent though caring profession to what we have today—a highly specialized, semi-scientific system. But the downside of this rapid expansion of knowledge is that health care practitioners now may experience deficiencies in the personal expression of the human elements of empathy: compassion and caring. How much of all this can be taught and then comprehended by the modern medical student? Surely, there is a danger of concentrating too much on how things work in the micro dimensions of life to the exclusion of how and why they work in the larger dimension of human activity in health and illness. When the growth in specialization and pharmaceutical agents is coupled with the growth in legal actions against physicians and the increasingly high cost of physician medical insurance, the reasons for the impersonal aspects of medical care come into a more realistic perspective. From all this comes the need for greater attention to the ethics involved, both for the big-ticket items (end of life issues such as euthanasia, resource allocation, informed consent, new reproductive choices) and the small-ticket ones (such as patient-practitioner trust, respect for people, friendship).

Of course, these advances in medical science did not happen in a vacuum; there were also great changes in the sociological aspects of health care and health delivery during this time. As health care became more effective, it became ethically more important that it should no longer be a privilege of the wealthy but a necessity for all, in recognition of the fundamental ethical principle of the moral equality of all in a given society. Adequate health care came to be seen as an entitlement based on this principle and society, for the first time in history, was prepared to finance it. In Britain, these social changes were modeled on a plan by British economist William Beveridge (1879–1963), which included the National Health Service (NHS), introduced in 1948. Hospitals became places where diseases were diagnosed and treated by the new class of specialists and not places where people went to die, as was the pattern in the 18th and 19th centuries.

There was also a change in the role of physicians during these various epochs of medicine. In 1666, when the plague hit London, the College of Physicians (representing London physicians) was accused of fleeing the capital. They justified themselves by saying that they left because all their patients had left. This was certainly true at that time because only the rich had physicians. Most people relied on nothing or the services of apothecaries.

The medical profession resisted the introduction of the NHS in post-War Britain, just as they would a decade or so later when Tommy Douglas introduced Medicare to Saskatchewan, and for the same reasons: self-interest, and distrust of bureaucracy and the fee schedule. But British doctors eventually bought into the plan. To many physicians, the terms of NHS service seemed fair, and even attractive, but others emigrated to Canada, Australia or the U.S. because they disliked the "capitation system," where each citizen is enrolled with a general practitioner, who in turn receives a fixed annual fee for looking after the health needs of this individual. This trend to state-supported health care later spread throughout Europe and most of the developed world, except the U.S. (aside from Medicaid and Medicare, which provide health care for the poor and elderly). Thus, it was during the third epoch that physicians began serving the entire populace.

By the end of the third epoch, health delivery had changed from something you either could or could not afford, something that was conducted in your own home by a visiting physician, or in his (the gender bias was almost absolute) office, into a publicly funded system where the hospital played a much larger role and women constituted half the medical profession. Through my own experiences as a physician, I have witnessed how the attitudes of physicians changed, how patients became better informed about their illnesses and aware of their entitlements, and how the potencies of new technologies (pharmaceutical, biological, physical and surgical) gave enormous power to effect good outcomes, but carried great potential to cause new and unexpected harms.

It is not surprising that the whole topic of health ethics came to life during this epoch, and then became increasingly important both to physicians (who perhaps were slow to understand how their world was changing) and to others (patients, administrators, lawyers, philosophers and those in pastoral care), and gave rise to a new breed of individual at the bedside—the bioethicist, accompanied by new backup systems such as Research Ethics Boards and Institutional Ethics Committees.

The expectation is that the **fourth epoch** (2000–2060) will see a flowering of medical measures based on genetics (see Appendix 2), genomics, and other aspects of molecular medicine.

One thing is certain: as medicine increases in complexity, so too will the ethical dilemmas. This is aptly illustrated by the early days of kidney dialysis* and the evolution of transplantation. During the 40 years I had the privilege of practicing nephrology and transplantation immunology, we gained much insight into the nature of kidney diseases and ways to control some of them, and grappled, practically from the outset, with complex ethical dilemmas.

In the early days of renal dialysis, when treatment cost about $25,000 (Canadian) per patient per year, medicine faced the difficult question of resource allocation: how much money and other resources should be spent to extend the lives of a small number of people, when the need elsewhere was so great? And given that dialysis was available in only a few centres, there was the related dilemma of selecting who received the treatment and who did not. It is no wonder that the nephrologists making these decisions at this time were referred to as belonging to "The God Squad."[5,6]

In addition to questions about resource allocation and patient selection, the advent of kidney transplantation raised more ethical quandaries that eventually spawned the whole discipline of transplantation ethics. Success in organ transplantation enormously increased the demand for organs and tissues, bringing with it such concepts as the recognition of brain criteria for determining death, the legal ability to decide on organ and tissue donation at one's death, "required request" or "presumed consent" of those dying with such criteria, and other related ethical issues.

The shortage of organs for human transplantation has also spawned the dilemma of whether human beings should be able to sell one of their two kidneys for personal gain—creating a human kidney market.[7] There is also the ethical question of whether financial incentive should be used to encourage families to donate the organs of loved ones who have died. Another dilemma is: how much of this research on the basic elements of human life should be patented by research outfits for their later profit?

---

* Dialysis is the process of cleaning wastes from the blood artificially. The blood travels through tubes to a dialyzer, which removes wastes and extra fluid. The cleaned blood then flows through another set of tubes back into the body. This job is normally done by the kidneys but if the kidneys fail, the blood must be cleaned artificially with special equipment. The two major forms of dialysis are hemodialysis and peritoneal dialysis.

It now looks as if the first decade of the new millennium, the fourth epoch, will see three trends in this field:

1. a refocusing on inducing immune tolerance in the recipient in contrast to the current search for more effective immune suppression for the recipient;
2. xenotransplantation or the use of animal organs as transplants into humans; and
3. attempts to grow vital tissues and organs from primitive cells, which retain their full potential to differentiate under appropriate stimuli. Such cells are known as toti-potential stem cells and there is a great surge of interest in this field.

Ethical debate is already raging in each of these three areas and, undoubtedly, new quandaries will surface in nephrology and medicine in general during the fourth epoch.

For me, this sea change in modern medicine began with Prof. Bulbring's accident and the experimental use of penicillin, and swept me through my entire career into nephrology, transplantation, research and medical ethics.

My first foray into research also involved another experimental use of penicillin in a clinical setting. In 1950—seven years after Prof. Bulbring's accident—I became the most junior member of a team at Bart's. We were trying to cure an infection of heart valves called subacute bacterial endocarditis (SBE)—an almost uniformly fatal condition. We gave large doses of penicillin in conjunction with another drug that cut down the urinary excretion of penicillin so as to build the blood levels of penicillin even higher. Patients with this condition were being sent from all over the U.K. to this unit in London. The organism was *Streptococcus viridans*, not a very penicillin-sensitive organism, especially when well tucked away in the fibrous tissue of a heart valve. But the cure rate with high doses of penicillin was very good.[8] Another disease had met its nemesis.

It was thrilling to be part of this innovation—a feeling that nothing quite matches. Rather than an immediate and fleeting thrill, my sense of satisfaction grew gradually and deepened with time. I have been fortunate to experience this on several occasions.

At the time, I did not think of the possible ethical concerns during this clinical research. In retrospect, however, I see that the new tool, penicillin, was so powerful that an uncontrolled trial was ethically appropriate; the known mortality rate of SBE served as historical controls. Indeed, in light of this fact, it would have been unethical to have used a control group of untreated patients.

But the fact remains that this potential to do great good also opened a window to the equal possibility of doing harm. And thus, not only did penicillin usher in a fantastic new era in therapeutics and a new epoch of medicine, it also increased the complexity and scope of ethical questions, which eventually came to dominate my career.

[A]s a young man, I used to try to picture in my imagination the feelings and ambitions of a white boy with absolutely no limit placed upon his aspirations and activities. I used to envy the white boy who had no obstacles placed in the way.... In later years, I confess that I do not envy the white boy as I once did. I have learned that success is to be measured not so much by the position that one has reached in life as by the obstacles which he has overcome while trying to succeed.

Booker T. Washington (1856–1915)
Up from Slavery: An Autobiography, 1901

2

Early medical career:
The student life and army experience

IN RETROSPECT, IT IS CURIOUS that I was neither aware of being on the cusp of great advances in medicine—except in a general sense—nor that my training was seriously deficient in the realm of ethics and moral philosophy. The student's life was crammed with facts to be learned and later reproduced in tests or more formal university examinations. The rest of one's time was spent frivolously in sport and amusement. It was a carefree life even though London was being bombed and battles were being fought in Libya, Italy, Normandy and the Pacific. World War II was part of everyone's experience, but being in a reserved category, I was not called upon for military service until 1951, by which time there was military action only in Malaya and, later, Korea.

My experience as a medical student consisted of two phases. From 1943–1945, I studied anatomy, physiology, pharmacology, biochemistry and organic chemistry at Oxford. Then from 1946–1949, I did my clinical training in medicine, surgery, pathology, bacteriology, psychiatry, radiology, obstetrics and gynecology at St. Bartholomew's Hospital, and took both the Oxford and London medical degrees in 1950.

It is arguably facile to find fault with the ethical aspects of my education and training against the backdrop of what we now hold to be ethical behaviour, but it is a useful measure of just how far we have progressed in such a relatively short period of time. Nowhere is this more aptly illustrated during my days as a medical student than during the obstetric rotation.

One of the aspects of medical student life towards which most of us looked with anticipation, tinged with trepidation, was the requirement to deliver 20 babies before graduation. This was not possible at Bart's because there simply were not enough normal deliveries among the dwindling inner-city population it served. Complicated cases were the prerogative of the house-staff (residents)* and there was no place for students, except as spectators. The humble medical student gained his or her experience by working with the midwives who performed deliveries in the district, which included areas such as Clerkenwell, Smithfield, Islington and other boroughs served by Bart's. (I say "his or her" because my class, the graduates of 1949, was the first in the hospital's 400-year history to have women students—seven in all.)

The expert knowledge during my rotation for obstetrics in December 1948 was almost entirely in the hands and heads of the district midwives. They were terrific, but the pregnant women who were being delivered at home on the National Health Service seemed to like having the medical students there. So, it seemed, did the grandmothers. I think they looked upon us as being well qualified; indeed, I suspect that most of them thought that we were real doctors, which we certainly were not.

I have vivid memories of riding a bicycle, obstetrical bag lashed to the back, to Clerkenwell Mansions, a large block of ten- or 12-storey tenement apartments with open-air staircases and no elevators. The name Mansions reflects the dignity and condescension of the philanthrope who endowed these tenements towards the end of the 19th century rather than the appearance of the building itself 50 years or so later.

Arriving on the appropriate floor, toting my bag of tricks, Peggy, the nurse-midwife, quickly indicated the mother's stage of labour. I had an immense respect for all the nurse-midwives I encountered, and Peggy was no exception, having delivered many hundreds of multiparous mums on the district. There was lots of brown paper on the floor, the light was dim and Granny was lurking in the background. Peggy knelt behind me and whispered in my ear: "Give that a firm hand!" "Don't stretch it. Squeeze it back over the occiput!" "Bring the legs up over her abdomen!" "Have the clamp ready; that's it, clamp it just about there but milk some blood out of the cord before you do." Thank goodness that every step was guided by her wonderful expertise. At the end, Granny said, "It was so

* The British term for an intern or resident, the period of training after completing medical school. After two or three years as a resident, doctors may choose to practise as a general practitioner or to specialize and train for another three to five years, depending on their specialty.

Ethical Dilemma

Such were the privileges of being a student. I should have said, "Thanks for your kind words, Ma'am, but please know that I am a student and not yet a real doctor. All the real expertise this evening rests with the nurse-midwife. Actually, Ma'am, this is only the third delivery I have ever seen, myself." I should have been open and honest about that aspect.

Later, much later, as a professor of health ethics, I would certainly give all students that advice. But, on that occasion, long ago, I indulged in the wonderful privileges that becoming a physician afforded a young man, albeit through a deception of imperfect disclosure. It was evidence of the innate paternalism of the medical mystique in those days, 50 years ago.

I was also quite conscious of this ongoing mild deception when I became a house-physician, a year or so later. I often wondered whether patients understood that I was learning the trade at the same time as I was offering professional services. Some did, but I suspect that most did not. The ethical goal should be appropriate disclosure—disclosure, but not in such a way as to completely undermine trust in the overall value of the supervised process. Did the workers at the Smithfield meat market, coming to emergency with gashes from their knives, know that the person suturing the gash might be a medical student or recent graduate who had never done it before? No, but they knew from years of experience that they would be taken care of at the hospital.

good to have you here, doctor; we know that nurse is very good, but it's good to have the doctor present as well."

"Thanks very much," I murmured, tacitly going along with the paternalistic posture.

"By the way, doctor, can I tempt you with a glass of sherry before you go?" she asked.

The rest of the obstetrical rotation was fairly trite in comparison to the experiences on the district, but one other memory involving myself and a student friend surges back. We were attending the Christmas party, where we had both had a beer or two, and maybe a glass of wine, when we were called to a delivery in the main hospital department, under

Ethical Dilemma

It would have been better if no drinking was permitted for those on call. But at Bart's in those days, with a pub across the road from the emergency department, and a beer bar downstairs in the residents' quarters, beer drinking was allowed—although the consumption of spirits definitely was not. It should be noted too, that British beer at that time had an alcohol content of only one to three per cent, and so a glass of beer was considered to be merely another beverage.

It is interesting to note that the pubs across the road from most London hospital emergency rooms played a historic role. Indeed, in the emergency room at Bart's, one could still see the leather strap markings on the arms of some of the hard wood and leather chairs where patients would be strapped down, plied with rum or gin, and then operated upon with considerable dexterity and speed. The anesthetic agent came from the pub, of course.

I must say that I never saw any serious breach of behaviour because of drinking on the wards or in the clinics, though that could not be said of the Saturday afternoon excursions by bus to the hospital's sports facilities at Chislehurst, Surrey. Returning from those adventures was usually rude, raucous and at times revolting!

The reason for not allowing residents on call to consume alcohol really comes down to the ethical issue of consent to adequate disclosure. Patients are entitled to assume that there is no possibility that those who attend them are under alcoholic influence. It might be acceptable, theoretically, if a resident who had had a drink or two were to make a point of letting each patient know this fact in the course of caring for him or her. But this would be so deleterious to that element of trust, which underpins all these relationships, as to render these relationships ineffective. Again, the absence of consent, following adequate disclosure, can be traced back to the inherent paternalism in medicine in those days. Let us never forget that age-old maxim: "Doctor knows best!"

experienced nurse supervision. My friend dexterously caught the baby and made off with her to the bassinet. There was an immediate tightening of the cord.

"Shouldn't you clamp and cut that thing, George," I said gently, trying to sound nonchalant.

"My God, how right you are, John," he exclaimed in return.

A junior nurse twittered nervously in the background.

I enjoyed obstetrics and worked quite hard at acquiring book knowledge. Soon afterwards I won the Matthew Duncan prize in Obstetrics. I even wondered if obstetrics should be my calling. But the real reason for my enthusiasm, I think, was that I had taken about six weeks off in the summer of 1948 to go to South Africa to play field hockey in an Oxford/Cambridge composite team called the Swallows and felt a bit guilty about it when I returned to take up my training in obstetrics, so I was determined to do well.

The Swallows tour was paid for by the South African teams, the state and the university. They did not feel they were up to Olympic standards of competition, but they spent the equivalent amount sponsoring a touring team while the 1948 Olympic Games were being held in London. This was wonderful for the 15 of us and we gave them a good run for their money on the field.

Of course, there was no question of meeting, let alone playing against, black African teams. Indeed, there was much talk of apartheid (from the Afrikaans word for "apartness") though the early political spokesman for that atrocious ideology was quite active as leader of the opposition party at the time. Everyone in 1948, however—every White, that is—was convinced that the future was good. We met Field Marshal Jan Smuts, then still prime minister, who emphasized the great opportunities central Africa presented for Englishmen and encouraged us to spend our careers there. Actually, two team members did just that, but I was keen to get back to my studies and was hoping I had not missed too much. Hence my dedication to obstetrics for the next few months after my return.

Postgraduate work

I graduated in medicine in January of 1950. A peculiar time of the year you might think, and you are right. Despite some prior claims to academic prowess, I was "ploughed" at the Oxford bachelor of medicine, bachelor of chirurgerie—or surgery—(BM, BCh) exams in December 1949, much to my chagrin and everyone's surprise. It would be tedious to recount all the reasons why I failed, but two factors seemed relevant to me at the time. First, there was my romantic involvement with young Dorothy Reid, a wonderful Bart's nurse with whom I had been spending a lot of time, and second, there was the intermittent toxicity and withdrawal effects of my indecisiveness and weak-minded control over nicotine. It seems almost ridiculous to claim this in retrospect, but there it is.

I had applied to work as a house-officer (or resident, as it is known in Canada) with Prof. Ronald V. Christie, Chief of the Medical Professorial Service at Bart's. I assumed I would start at the beginning of January after graduating in December. When I failed the Oxford exams I let the chief know of my disappointment. "Don't let that bother you," he advised. "Pass the London exams and come on my service at the end of January instead." For a young man who was down at the time, this was a gesture for which I will always be grateful. He did more for me later, but this first encounter made me his man for life.

In early January I passed the London Membership of the Royal College of Physician (MRCP) and Licentiate of the Royal College of Surgeons (LRCS) exams. I began working as a junior house-physician at Bart's on February first, one month late, but as promised, Prof. Christie had kept a position open for me because these posts are more or less continuous work. I did not have a chance to do any book revision for the Oxford examinations in June 1950, but I was truly fortunate on this second throw and earned both my bachelors of medicine and chirurgerie.

At that time in England, medical graduates spent one year as a junior house-officer, followed by two years as a senior house-officer, after which they could become a general practitioner, or go on to become a specialist or consultant as a junior then senior registrar—a process that took another two or three years.

It was while serving as junior house-officer on the professorial service[*] for the rest of 1950 that I was exposed to my first taste of clinical research. As mentioned in the previous chapter, the project was to find out if penicillin worked on a condition of infection of the heart valves called

---

[*] In the London teaching hospitals, there was usually one professor of medicine. The other services were headed by attending consultants with rooms in Harley Street. They were equal to the professor, but they did not enjoy University of London academic appointments; nor did they want them, because such appointments would have considerably reduced their incomes.

subacute bacterial endocarditis, which, though rare, was 100 per cent fatal at that time. Later, the work was published in the *Quarterly Journal of Medicine*[9] (without mention of the humble house-officers, of course) and was heralded as a significant advance in the management of this condition.

I have particularly pleasant memory of spending Christmas at the hospital. Though my father had just died, unexpectedly, in November and I had spent a few days at home in Bromham, Wiltshire, the entertainment of patients at Christmas was a must, and I returned to it as a means of getting over my grief at losing my life's best counsellor. In those days, no student or house-officer thought of going home if they were involved in their group's Christmas show. It was a tradition. A tradition, I might add, which involved the audience—the people from that part of London who considered Bart's part of their life. I recall one old dear's disappointment when I said, "That's all, now, Mrs. Jenkins—I will see you in mid-January." "You mean you are not going to admit me to the hospital for Christmas, Doc?" she asked. "I haven't missed a Christmas in there since me old man passed away—it's always such a hard time of year for my baronichals, doc!" (She had longstanding bronchiectasis, a chronic inflammation in the lung's bronchioles.) I relented, of course. After all, she was more part of the place than I was, and the National Health Service was in its youthful heyday.

The festivities included the house-officers developing a musical skit with songs about contemporary ward and medical school characters. We, and the other firms, went around the wards performing our show for several days during that holiday period, a time of great merriment and glee.

Many others have written about being a junior house-physician—it is a fascinating indoctrination process into the medical world that entails exceedingly long hours, more responsibility than one should have and learning the craft at an enormous pace. We made mistakes and had small triumphs; all of life's pathos was condensed and magnified during these years. A few poignant incidents stand out from the routines of ward rounds, emergency admissions and clinics.

The first involved my mistakenly giving an intravenous injection of an iron compound to a 55-year-old man who was sitting on a chair by his bed. He fainted on me (a vaso-vagal syncope) and finished up on the floor of the ward with my needle in his arm. Fortunately, he came round within a few moments. It caused a commotion in the 36-bed ward; he made quite a clatter and I blushed with shame.

The second incident involved giving an attractive, asthmatic young woman injections of her own blood (called auto-hemotherapy) into the buttock muscles on orders of the registrar. After I was through, he sniggered: "Did you get a kick out of doing that, John?" I thought it was a crudely inappropriate and unprofessional comment. That particular medical practice was later discontinued as being totally useless, anyway.

Third, I injected morphine subcutaneously (under the skin) to a man who was labouring mightily to breathe with long-standing severe emphysema (a bubble-like transformation of the lungs that interferes with oxygen uptake). First his breathing eased, then he turned from being grateful to being tranquil, and in 20 minutes he ceased breathing and died. There was much discussion and no resolution, except for myself; I vowed never to repeat such a treatment. Did I kill him? The thought seemed inescapable. I was very disturbed, although my seniors did their best to point out his hopeless prognosis and terminal state. Still, that memory lingers to this day. It was the first time I realized how easy it is, in caring for others who are so very weakened and vulnerable, to do them harm rather than good.

The fourth incident involved being responsible for a dying man in his 30s who had a lymphosarcoma (a cancer of the cells that are responsible for the body's immunity) of the stomach that had spread to the liver and had eroded into the colon. He was past any point where surgery might help. He was agonized by fecal vomiting—a very unpleasant condition, where the contents of his large bowel (the transverse part of the colon) escaped back into his stomach, causing him to vomit feces. The registrar said, "Dossetor, I don't expect to see that man tomorrow when I come on rounds. Do something!" It was my first experience of a situation where no treatment can offer benefit and one feels obligated to help the sufferer by relieving him by the only possible effective route. Certainly he was asking for relief; it did not matter how or what. He was given increasing doses of morphine and expired early next morning. One grows up under such conditions!

In this way, as a junior member of the hospital staff, I became much more aware that there was right and wrong in terms of medical conduct and, thereafter, such questions began to roil around my mind. But there did not seem to be any true opportunity to discuss these ethical dilemmas. Indeed, the term "ethical dilemma" would not have been understood by myself or my colleagues. Clearly one knew what it was to do good and to avoid doing wrong, but discussions of the sorts of dilemmas such as

Ethical Dilemma

What about the ethics of the four instances quoted above? Even now, years later, they are vivid memories that give me pause to think. Examined more closely, they clearly fall into four categories.

1. **An error.** It is a medical error to give an intravenous injection to someone who is sitting because if that person has even a short panic reaction there is a risk if falling off the chair. In fact, it is unethical not to think ahead to *all* the complications that could attend a medical action.

2. **An intimate action that might be wrongly thought to have sexual implications.** This aspect of medicine is inevitable when one considers the trust that female patients habitually show, and are expected to show, towards male practitioners. The practitioner must not only act appropriately, from a sexual standpoint, but must also be seen to act in an appropriate fashion, both by the female patient and by others who may be witnesses. The standard way of counteracting this risk is to ask a nurse or female medical student or intern to be present when an intimate examination or procedure is undertaken. Unfortunately, this is not always possible. It is also a simple fact that such situations can occur whenever men and women interact in almost every professional encounter or undertaking. The difference in the medical therapeutic or investigative situation is due to the greater vulnerability of the person whose psyche is more exposed and the consequent need for a greater degree of trust on the patient's part, and of integrity on the part of the practitioner.

3. **The importance of truly informed consent.** Injecting morphine into those with great shortness of breath has always had a risk. It was never clear to me why the initial improvement and gratitude was then followed by his death. Was the dose too great? Should it have been administered more slowly by a measured infusion? Were there other measures that might have helped? Did I consult sufficiently with those who had greater experience who were, theoretically, available to me? The example illustrates, in retrospect, the uncertainty surrounding the practice of

medicine. Every patient is unique and presents a unique problem. One can never presume that what should happen, will happen. There are many, many situations where uncertainty remains, even after full analysis. The uniqueness of each individual in reacting to what one hopes are actions in their best interest stresses the importance of truly informed consent.

4. **Active euthanasia.** In this case, I was faced with the dilemma of whether to relieve unbearable suffering even though it meant shortening life, albeit with the individual's knowing and understanding. My actions, in the case of this man with fecal vomiting, will be controvertible to many. He could have been left with his distress with lesser doses of morphine. He would surely have died within a few days of aspiration pneumonia from inhaled feces. This is not the place to go into a long discussion of relief of distress in the face of inevitable death, even though life might be shortened, as was the case here. Nor will I go into the question of the moral difference between withdrawal and withholding of treatment. A vital part of such situations involves communication with the patient and family, leading to comprehended choice. On both those scores my conscience is clear. But let no one pretend that there are simple ethical rules governing such tragic clinical situations.

Taken together, these examples illustrate the wide variety of ethical issues that occur in the practice of medicine and also the role of casuistry (resolving difficult ethical problems with clever but often false reasoning) in trying to understand them. It is difficult to approach them from a point of principle; nor are they completely covered by the themes that characterize the ethics of relationships. Later, I will expound further on the synthesis of these two approaches as the means—in a sort of dialectic analysis— that I have found to be most helpful in attempting to grapple with the ethics of other clinical situations. But the fact is that in the past, house-officers often had to face such problems without any formal training in medical ethics.

"quality of life" versus "sanctity of life" and its preservation at all costs, simply never occurred. Medical ethics, in those days, was not a recognized subject, except for vague understandings about the importance of the doctor-patient relationship. As will become apparent later, even such matters as obtaining fully informed consent were never adequately debated. The process at that juncture could better be described as obtaining perfunctory consent. I was later, much later, to learn that there were codes of ethics, including ethics in medical research.

Training in cardiology

At this point in my training I was interested in virtually every aspect of medicine. Obstetrics held me for a while and I considered psychiatry, then Dr. Graham Hayward, a cardiologist and second in command on the Bart's medical professorial unit, suggested I try cardiology. At his suggestion, I obtained a position as house-officer at the country branch of the National Heart Hospital at Maids Moreton, near Buckingham, 80 km (50 miles) from the main National Heart Hospital in central London. The job also entailed spending two days a week in London, taking calls for the house-officer there.

I had a feeling of real responsibility for the 50 or so convalescent heart patients at Maids Moreton, and enjoyed it. One particular friend was little Wendy, a ten-year-old with longstanding heart failure, whose tense protuberant abdomen had to be tapped for ascitic fluid every two to three weeks. Although she was a long-stay patient at the heart hospital, she was also my friend and I took her almost everywhere in my car as I drove around Buckinghamshire, though I was careful to make sure that the nursing Sister knew where she would be. The other was Rajah, our stolid loveable Elkhound—almost human in every way—whom I took everywhere, including on ward rounds, having trained him to go under the bed when Sister appeared.

During this training, I decided I wanted to become a cardiologist and certainly, at these two locations, had every opportunity to see a vast range of heart disease (mainly of the chronic variety and much of it chronic rheumatic heart disease), and to meet the leading London cardiologists of the day.

A personal dilemma

I had been medically examined for army service at intervals after having been in a reserved category while a medical student at Oxford and at Bart's. In 1948, a shadow was found at the central area (hilum) of my lungs, which was diagnosed as the mediastinal lymph node enlargement of Boerck's sarcoidosis—a relatively benign condition. Two years later the glands were smaller. The radiologist offered me the choice, essentially, of remaining in a non-service category for several more years, or of being declared fit for service immediately. I was tempted to opt for the former course so I could begin shaping my career as a specialist (cardiologist, as I then supposed), but it also was a challenge of conscience. After a couple of days, I called back to say I wanted the clean bill of health. He agreed, and so it was.

Within three months, I was sent a notice to report to the Royal Army Medical Corps training barracks in Aldershot for basic training. Square bashing—marching up and down the square carrying a rifle—under the eye of regular sergeants could not be described as fun, but the collegiality made it worthwhile. After several weeks, a half-colonel came down from London to brief us on possible postings. He said the War Office wanted to disrupt our career plans as little as possible so I told him of my ambition for specialist training in internal medicine and he said they would try to accommodate that. I was thus very surprised when my initial posting was to Singapore General Hospital. This was not at all what I had been expecting in the light of his assurances, and I voiced my disapproval. In front of the group, I told the half-colonel that I had no objection to where I would be sent, but thought it very inappropriate for him to have promised minimum career dislocation when he clearly did not have that authority. There was an embarrassing pause, but the moment soon passed.

A few weeks later I was on embarkation leave before going to the Far East, and decided that there was nothing I could do about it. But halfway through that leave period, I received a telegram saying: "Your posting changed. You will report to AMD7 [War Office Army Medical Department 7], Berkeley Square, London, next Thursday, at 08:00 hours."

Clearly they thought Dossetor was someone who needed closer watching! I found myself working on files of medical board findings from different theatres of army operations all over the world, and answering certain complaints about army life that involved health matters. At first I thought this might give me the freedom I wanted to work at other things, but it soon dawned on me that the prospect of serving out my two years at that sort of desk job was stultifying in the extreme. I remember one mother wrote that her son had feet of two different sizes and the army would only issue boots in pairs of the same size. Dossetor took care of that. There were also crackpot letters to the Queen that were routed through the office if they chiefly concerned medical matters, but not if they were in any way threatening to her person. Still, the monotony of AMD7 was soul-destroying.

Relief came my way in the course of a few weeks. By asking around, I found out who really made the postings for newly-conscripted medical officers. As anyone with true experience of the military knows, the senior non-commissioned officers really run things. (I have since found out that that is the way all organizations run; always look for the senior admin person if you really want to get things changed in a hurry. It is a principle that is certainly true in large hospitals.)

Using this piece of intelligence, I invited the appropriate AMD7 sergeant-major to share a few beers with me at the Colony restaurant in Berkeley Square and told him of my discontent.

He asked: "Well, where do you want to go?"

"As far away from the War Office as possible," I replied.

"Well, let me think for a moment. I can send you to the Caribbean as lieutenant, but how about this one? I could send you to the Nepalese border with India, to a recruiting camp for Ghurkha soldiers for the Far East forces in Singapore. You would go as an acting major, as you would be the senior of three British medical officers stationed in India. They are both conscripts, like you, you know. That is all we have in that vast country these days."

"Done," I said, "and have another drink, Sergeant-Major!"

India, 1951–1952

I welcomed this chance to go to India as a sort of homecoming. I was born in 1925 in Bangalore, India, while my parents were in the midst of a 20-year stint of service in that country. My father was an Anglican priest with the Indian Ecclesiastical Establishment, part of the British Raj, serving military communities. Three children were born during World War I. The second son, Peter, died in India in 1923 after being bitten by a rabid dog. My heartbroken parents had another child, Andrew in 1926, then realized that Andrew was eight years younger than his two remaining siblings and needed a companion. That is where I came in!

We lived in Bangalore, about halfway between Bombay and Madras, for two years, then moved to Belgaum for another three years. I have no particular memories of this time because at the age of five, I was sent with my three siblings to school in England. There, we boarded with a foster family and visited my father's friends during school holidays. Every year my parents would come to visit for a few months, and once, when I was eight and my brother Andrew was nine, we spent six months in India. At that time, my parents lived in Kirkee, a suburb of Pune and although we had never been to the house, it felt like home. I retain many memories of that time, in particular, riding ponies all over the place. My father retired from India in 1938 to become a country parson in England.

My father, an Australian who went to Britain for theological training at Wells Theological College, Somerset, in 1913, was not a jingoistic imperialist in any sense. Neither he nor my mother, also an Australian, ever completely bought the concept of the virtuous Empire upon "which the sun never set." However, my dad believed in the natural good that would come to the Indians from prolonged contact with a benign imperial power's culture, knowledge, technology, and, yes, even their religion. Though not a missionary himself, he was friendly with many missionaries of various denominations. While having an admiration for Mahatma Ghandi, he more or less shared then-prime minister Winston Churchill's description of the Mahatma as a "half-naked fakir" who caused trouble, and he doubted if India would survive as a democracy if given independence, especially if the subcontinent was split into Hindu and Muslims states.

As evidence of this, I recall my dad's conviction at the beginning of World War II that one of the best careers for me would be to enter the Sudanese civil service, and serve there until retirement. He thought the Sudan would be a better choice than India because of the greater likelihood of civil unrest in the India of the future. World War II changed all that sort of speculation, but recalling those attitudes may give a quick conceptual vignette of how the world seemed to an experienced man of the Anglican cloth who, in 1939, had three sons and a daughter to plan for.

For my generation, the incredible upheaval of World War II finished the idea of British imperialism. The empire was bankrupt; America and the USSR had taken over as the World powers. Empire clearly was an idea that was no longer sustainable, though many, my father included, believed that the new order would turn out to be regrettable for the undeveloped world. If alive today, he would likely point to sub-Saharan Africa and say, "See what I mean?"

The Raj ended in 1947, thus the India of my childhood was changing, but it was during my military service that I really cemented my relationship with the country. A month after my drink with the sergeant-major, I boarded a ship at Southampton for a three-week sea voyage to Bombay, followed by a train trip across central India to Calcutta to see one of my units at the army staging post. I then travelled back across Northern India, spending two nights on the train, and finishing with a trip of 70 km (40 miles) by jeep over dusty roads to the camp at Lehra, some 8 km (5 miles) from the border of India and Nepal, roughly in the middle of India. The Himalayas, dominated by mighty Mount Kanchanjunga, were clearly visible on days when there was no heat haze.

The life at Lehra was a curious one, as we lived half in the past. The old Raj was very much in evidence even though India was in its fourth year of independence and I, for one, thought the new mood and atmosphere in India was progressive and liberating. But, strange to relate, the Indian population in Lehra's neighbouring villages still felt that Britain was concerned for their welfare. I remember several villagers bringing disputes over property, dowries and the like to the officer's mess in search of a just solution and being quite stupefied when told that the Queen's government could no longer be an authority to which they could turn. It seemed as if no one had told them about independence; either that, or they did not really believe it.

The British army in India consisted only of two Ghurkha Brigade recruiting camps and a staging camp. Our presence was allowed there courtesy of the Indian government, though we were not meant to wear full uniform in public places. I found I was replacing a medical officer who had become too fond of gin. He had left before I arrived, but the other six officers welcomed me into their circle. The commanding officer, adjutant, paymaster, quartermaster and transport officer were regular British Ghurkha officers hoping for long service with their regiments. Three had served in World War II and two were more recently commissioned. In contrast, the other medical officer and I were national service draftees, serving two years and not committed in any way to the military life or the cult of the Ghurkha.

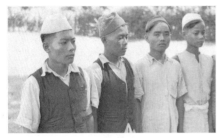

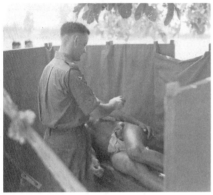

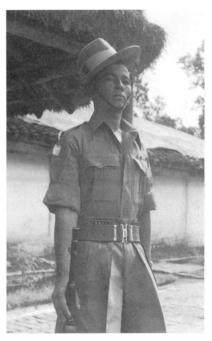

Four men from the valley of Nepal seeking careers in a Ghurkha regiment (top left). Recruits were assessed for fitness. Here a medical officer percusses for an enlarged spleen (bottom left). They all aspire to look like this eventually (right).

We led an interesting life, surrounded by 300 or so Ghurkha soldiers and their families living in tented accommodations, with recruits swelling the camp population at times, and parties of soldiers, in transit, on discharge, or on leave between Nepal and Singapore.* We had fairly good medical supplies, a 30-bed tented hospital, and a staff of Anglo-Indian nurses and orderlies (offspring of British soldiers and Indian women from 200 years of colonialism).

Much of the medical work was routine, but there were some high moments. The care of the soldiers did not provide a great challenge because, broadly speaking, they were very fit. The same could not be said of the local Indian villagers who had no medical services whatsoever. As a gesture of good will, after finishing the military sick parade that ran from 6:00 to 8:00 a.m., we conducted a second sick parade for any villager

---

* This was before the Korean War when Britain still controlled Singapore and Malaya (but not Burma). The communist insurrection came from the jungles bordering Thailand. Their infiltration into Malaya was resisted by Commonwealth troops based in Kuala Lumpur or Singapore, an important contingent of which was the British Brigade of Ghurkhas.

BEYOND THE HIPPOCRATIC OATH

Table 2.1   Initial diagnoses of 100 consecutive cases in the local Indian population, British Ghurkha Brigade Camp, Lehra, Uttar Pradesh, July 1953.

Affliction	Diagnosis	Number of cases
Acute fever		**6**
	malaria—malarial parasites seen	1
	kala-azar—clinical diagnosis only	1
	unknown cause	4
Large liver and spleen	chronic malaria or chronic kala-azar	**12**
Gastrointestinal		**15**
	clinical amoebiasis, many with hepatic tenderness	13
	acute bacillary dysentery (presumptive)	1
	haemorrhoids	1
Lung disease		**11**
	pulmonary tuberculosis (4 AFB-positive)	6
	asthma	1
	chronic productive cough (? TB or bronchiectasis)	3
	pleuritic pain (? cause)	1
Venereal disease	gonococcal demonstrable (1 vulva ulcer)	**8**
Urinary system		**4**
	cystitis	3
	type 1 nephritis	1
Cardiovascular		**2**
	? rheumatic fever	1
	chronic rheumatic valvular disease	1
Obstetrical		**2**
	fetal head retained in utero	1
	post-partum urinary incontinence	1
Eye disease		**3**
	conjunctivitis	2
	abscess on cornea	1
Otolaryngeal		**6**
	epiphora in an infant	1
	sinusitis	1
	acute mastoiditis	1
	discharging middle ears	2
	foreign body in ear	1
Skin diseases		**7**
	severe fungus disease of Langerhans cell granulomatosis	1
	erysipelas in an infant	1
	unknown cause	5
	pustular eruption of face and scalp of children	3

Affliction	Diagnosis	Number of cases
Leprosy		3
	eczema (? etiology)	2
	unknown cause	1
Neurological	peripheral neuritis	2
Sepsis		3
Ischio-rectal abscess		1
	septic palm	1
	flexor sheath infection of hand	1
Dental sepsis		3
	carious teeth extracted	2
	1 alveolar abscess	1
Trauma		2
Colles fracture		1
	fracture mid-femur (young boy)	1
Snake bite	patient died; said to be a cobra	1
Cancer	Epithelioma of the jaw	1
Unclassified		9
	2 headaches, no fever	2
	3 vague abdominal pains	3
	? depression	4
Total		**100**

who was sitting under the shade of certain tree adjacent to my tent at 9:00 in the morning.

The variety of their diseases was incredible (see Table 2.1). We figured that we had the world's highest proportion of visceral kala-azar, a severe infectious disease marked by fever, progressive anemia, leukopenia and enlargement of the spleen and liver. It is caused by leishmaniasis, a parasite, that is transmitted by sandfly bites. There was also much open tuberculosis (easily diagnosed from Ziehl-Nielsen staining of sputum under the microscope), malaria, malnutrition, leprosy, rabies, and the occasional outbreak of cholera.

We also had an operating room. As crude and poorly equipped though it was, it was the only one for tens of miles in any direction. I look back on that tented compound as the place that first engendered my concerns to understand more about medical ethics.

Some glimmers of medical ethics
Although all the offices, as well as the hospital, were housed in tents, the operating room was a Nissen hut with the operating room (OR) at one

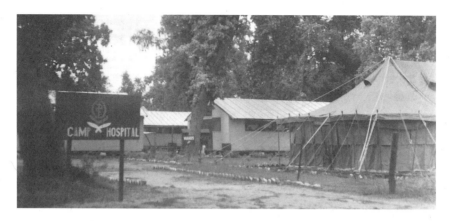

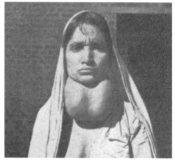

Camp Hospital (above), Lehra Depot at Uttar Pradesh, India, in 1952. Woman with goitre (right) and symptoms of tracheal obstruction at night.

end and store room at the other. I will describe two surgical experiences, though we had many. One is tragic, the other joyful.

In the first, the other medical officer and I decided to try and relieve obstruction to breathing being experienced by a woman with the largest goitre that I have ever seen (See photograph above). That part of the Himalayan foothills had very little iodine in the water, so goitre was endemic. This goitre was the size of a honeydew melon fitted under her chin. She came, or rather was brought, to us because there had been a recent increase in size and it was tender, presumably from a hemorrhage into part of it. She said, through interpreters—but one could never be sure that my interpreter understood the local Indian dialect—that she choked occasionally when sleeping.

We decided to operate though we knew there was a risk in doing so without blood transfusion support. Neither of us had any proper surgical training, though we could both give simple anesthesia. The operation was much more complicated than either of us realized. We got into progressive bleeding complications that we could not stanch. Things went fairly rapidly from bad to worse, and her tissues oozed and oozed. We tried to tie off all bleeding points but it did not seem to slow the bleeding. Her blood pressure slipped. Her pulse became barely detectable in the neck and she died on the operating table. Obviously, we felt terrible about this. The villager family took it as fate, I suppose, though our ability to communicate with them was limited. We wondered if we were doing the right thing in trying to provide medical service to these people.

One effect of this shattering experience was to force us to develop a blood transfusion service. The next day, I explained our problem to the Subadhur Major (the Indian equivalent to sergeant-major), asking him if it would be possible to ask for volunteer blood donors among the soldiers who staffed the depot (not soldiers in transit because we had no blood storage facility). We could then determine their blood groups (a simple slide agglutination test) and call them when we needed them to donate blood. He saluted smartly and replied "Huzoor!", his eyes seemingly riveted on the distant horizon. We hoped he had understood what we wanted.

The next morning, there were staccato shouted orders and the thumping of boots just a few metres from my tent. The Subadhur Major came in under the tent flap and announced that the volunteers were outside. I ducked out and there were all the Ghurkha soldiers of the camp drawn up in rows. "Have they all volunteered?" I asked, somewhat naïvely. He saluted smartly and said "Huzoor!" This time there was a glint in his eye! So we blood-typed them all and thereafter the depot had a volunteer blood bank, on the hoof as it were, for use with future surgery.

A month or so later we had need of them. A young woman (about 15 or 16, though her age was difficult to guess) who had been in labour

Ethical Dilemma

What of the old Hippocratic statement *Primum non nocere*: First, do no harm? How long would she have lived if we had done nothing? How much of our motivation was enthusiasm to do something to save a threatened life and how much was to see if we could meet this challenge to our medical prowess—a form of seemingly justified irresponsibility? Certainly there was no informed consent in the usual sense of those words, for three main reasons: we could not fully inform her of the risk because we did not know; we did not discuss alternative courses of action; and we did not disclose our own inexperience. All cardinal aspects of informed consent.

for several days was brought in late one night. On examining her we found that there was a round object in the lower abdomen, which seemed to be the head of a full grown fetus, but we could not palpate other fetal body parts. It transpired that she had gone into a breech presentation, but the body had been pulled off the head, leaving the head in the uterus. There was bleeding and shock, and the vulva was soiled by various sticky salves that had been applied by the village women who had attended her.

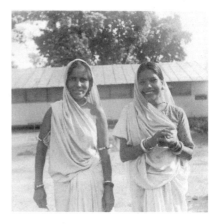

The patient who underwent a Caesarean section at a follow-up visit, accompanied by her mother.

Taking out the fetal head, by then very probably infected, through the lower anterior abdominal wall incision put her at considerable risk of an awful infection. We both deemed that leaving her alone would have been much worse. We called up two appropriately-typed blood donors and an orderly took their blood into sterile plastic bags and hung them up. My colleague gave the anesthesia and I rapidly performed my first and last Caesarean section. I then admitted her to the hospital, gave her penicillin and sulphonamide drugs and hoped for the best. In fact, she did just fine, and was taken home by her family several days later.

During my remaining six months there, every morning when I went down to my tent at 6:00 A.M. there was little pile of scented flowers on the corner of the desk: frangipani, jasmine and the like. I never saw who put them there and the soldier/orderly had no idea where they came from, or so he said.

Out of India

After about 18 months in Lehra, it was time for me to leave. I was ordered to deliver a report on my charge to my boss, a brigadier at the British Military Hospital in Singapore, which was still a British possession. I went on a grain ship from Calcutta, through Rangoon and Kuala Lumpur, to Singapore. After reporting, I spent most of the next week sailing at the Singapore Yacht Club, which was a wonderful, though solitary, experience. I had a strong urge to see some more of the East, so I

Ethical Dilemma

One may have to balance *Primum non nocere* against "high risks that may have to be accepted when there are no safer alternatives and life is threatened." At least there was no problem with lack of informed consent in this instance; it was clear to the family and the young woman what was wrong and that something had to be done to clear the uterus. We elected not to spend time explaining that the man about to do the Caesarean section had not done one before, though he had seen them done by others.

obtained leave to go on a troop ship that was leaving Singapore with British troops for Korea, via Hong Kong. There was no trouble adding me to the medical officers already on board as an extra medical hand. I little dreamed that I would have to do anything.

Two evenings out there was a storm, during which a soldier reported sick with acute abdominal pain. There were three medical officers on board: the regular ship's surgeon, another national service medical officer and myself. The regular ship's surgeon was drunk, so the pair of junior medical officers had to do something. Fortunately, my companion had done a year as a surgical house-officer. I gave the anesthesia; he operated. The ship was pitching and tossing about and the operating table was moving likewise, making surgery so hazardous that we had to call the bridge and ask the skipper to head directly into the storm for an hour, so that we could finish the job of removing this soldier's appendix. The skipper complied and that steadied things a bit. Yes, the appendix was acutely inflamed. Thank God, all went well. We felt pretty pleased with our inexperienced selves. A day or so later we put him off in the British Medical Hospital at Hong Kong, and I visited him the next day. He was doing fine.

My last medical exploit in the military was much less distinguished. As a national serviceman on discharge, I was put in medical charge of 40 or so soldiers who were also due for discharge en route back to England. We travelled by day in a large barely-furnished transport plane with very uncomfortable temporary seats. As I recall, we spent the first night at Calcutta, the next at Karachi, the third at Bahrain, the last at Cyprus. On the last night but one, one of the young British soldiers complained of earache and fever. I had a look at him and could see nothing much wrong. His ear was inflamed, as was his throat; the light in the barracks was poor and I did not notice anything else. We took him with us as far as Cyprus, but on arrival there his earache was worse, especially during take-off and landing. I decided that he should be put off the flight and thought that was the end of the matter.

Arriving at an army airport north of London the next day, the plane was surrounded by ambulances and Red Cross vehicles. Clearly, the army was flapping. It seems that the medical people in Cyprus diagnosed my patient as having measles. I had missed it. The enanthem (an internal eruption on mucous surfaces, such as the mouth and the back of the throat) must have been causing the earache and I had missed the exanthem (rash) on his body altogether. I can easily recall this, only to relive my chagrin. However, I was leaving the army next day and this diagnostic blooper on my part has not been fully revealed or admitted to the rest of the world, until now.

I could not afford to brood about this mistake because I was stressed by the more pressing question: "What on earth comes next?" I was at a new starting point in my career, though I managed first to put together my medical experiences as my first publication in medical literature. The paper, "Village practice on the Ganges plain," appeared in the *St Bartholomew's Hospital Medical Journal*[10] in April 1954.

A contemporaneous advance in science

During my absence, medicine had taken a giant leap forward. Just as my experience as a medical officer in an outpost of a dying Empire represented the end of a political era, so the discovery of the double helical structure of DNA by James Watson (1928–) and Francis Harry Compton Crick (1916–2004) heralded a new era—the third epoch—of medical science (see Appendixes 1 and 2). From this discovery emerged all of our knowledge about how genes regulate the function of cells and body organs, and the way that cells turn on or off the generation of enzymes. It would take several decades for this remarkable discovery to show its significance in terms of patient care, but that period of imaginative and informed thinking would prove to be for the 20th century what Darwin's theory of evolution had been for the 19th. (For anyone who wants to relive the romance of that epic discovery, I warmly recommend Watson's short but epic book, *The Double Helix*.[11] Years later,

Ethical Dilemma

This was my first experience of a situation that often faces physicians: how severe should one be on the misbehaviours of one's fellow physicians? The ship's doctor was too intoxicated to handle the abdominal emergency and we should have reported him to the medical command at Singapore. We assumed that the ship's captain, who was responsible for the discipline of all those on board, would know about this and act on his own. But that posture is really no more than a cop-out. We were two-year draftees and really very insignificant in the broad sweep of things, whereas the ship's surgeon had two or three decades of service. But the fact remains that he was incapable of acting in the care of the many men being transported to fight in Korea. The reader will find it hard to condone our passivity, and indeed, so do I. This was only the first of a number of instances during my career when I was faced with bad behaviour by a professional colleague. I like to think that I gained some integrity in such matters later on.

I made it, along with a companion gem, *In Defense of the Body*,[12] compulsory reading for anyone taking up work in the laboratory of the Medical Research Council Transplant Group in Alberta.)

What of ethics?

Despite this glimmer of the future of medical science, medical ethics was largely undiscovered and unfathomable in the early 1950s. Medical knowledge endows one with a power and a responsibility to practise for the good of others, but the idea that the vulnerable sick had an active role to play in these decisions was alien. Consent to treatment, of course! But fully informed consent? Never heard of it. The traditional paternalism of the professional, shared with priests, lawyers, the officer class in the military, and imperial administrators, was alive and well in most branches of public life—all of which were dominated by men.

Medical ethics, though never talked about, was subsumed, on the one hand, by the concept of commitment to patient care and a willingness to put that patient interest before one's own interests in the doctor-patient relationship—what the contemporary medical ethicist Albert R. Jonsen[13] has called the legacy of medieval monasticism and Knights Hospitallers of the Crusades era.* On the other hand, there was a commitment to competence based on knowledge of disease§ and the avoidance of doing harm, within a strong ethos of paternalism—the Hippocratic idea†—fuelled by the idea (never actually expressed) that doctor knows best.

As will be discussed later, these attitudes changed radically in the profession of medicine by the end of the millennium, but the change was not precipitous and certainly had not taken place during the year and a half that I spent in India in the early 1950s. Indeed, they did not really start to change until my emigration to Canada in 1955.

---

* The Benedictine rule stated that "the care of the sick is to be placed above and before every other duty." Those who cared for the sick, in these medieval traditions, were instructed to be servants to "our lords, the sick."

§ "Conclusions that are merely words cannot bear fruit, but only those based on demonstrated fact.... One must hold fast to generalizable fact and occupy oneself with facts persistently, if one is to acquire that ready and sure habit which we call the art of medicine...for to do so will bestow great benefit upon the sick."
—Hippocrates, precepts 2.

† "I will act for the benefit of my patient according to my ability and judgment and do no harm or injustice [to] lessen the violence of disease, relieve pain and avoid attempts to cure those whom disease has overcome."
—Hippocrates

LIZA: Will you drop me altogether now that the experiment is over, Colonel Pickering?

PICKERING: Oh don't. You mustn't think of it as an experiment. It shocks me, somehow.

LIZA: Oh, I'm only a squashed cabbage leaf—but I owe so much to you that I should be very unhappy if you forgot me....I was brought up to be just like him, [Professor Higgins], unable to control myself, and using bad language on the slightest provocation. And I should never have known that ladies and gentlemen didn't behave like that if you hadn't been there....

George Bernard Shaw (1856–1950)
Pygmalion (1916)

3

Two postgraduate years in London:
A lesson in patient vulnerability

IN 1954 I WAS FINISHED WITH THE ARMY and as I had no responsibilities apart from my widowed mother, I moved in with her in London. I began looking around for an opportunity, but training positions were few and far between because of the great influx of potential trainees from all over the Commonwealth and the U.S. I wanted to enter cardiology, but I had few contacts, and like many such things in life, it is often a question of whom one knows. Fortunately, I had my long-time Oxford friend, Dr. Bill Summerskill (who went on to head the gastrointestinal unit at the Mayo Clinic). A month or so after I came home, he suggested that I apply for further training as a resident in medicine at the Royal Post-Graduate Medical School in Hammersmith, West London, where he was also working. The position was part of a clinical research unit dedicated to liver disease and proudly sailed under the flag of the somewhat daunting Dr. (Dame) Sheila Sherlock—later to be recognized worldwide as the Queen of the Liver. Physicians, professors and postgraduates from all over the globe flocked to sit at her feet, or rather, to trail around behind her on ward rounds—the thrice-weekly parade.

I jumped at the chance to work with her; it was not cardiology, but it would allow me to carry on developing a subspecialty in internal medicine. Sherlock told me, on the day I joined for a nine-month training period, that I would be responsible for everything that happened to the patients, seven days a week and every weekend. If I chose to take time off because work was light, I should know that I was still responsible for the patients on both wards, even while I was out of the building. She also told me part of my job was to protect the liver failure patients from the scientific zeal of her registrars and research fellows. "They are vulnerable people, you know," she said. I took that as more or less a joke at the time. I will later relate how inadequate I now think my watch over the patients' welfare really was.

As junior on that service, in the face of gruelling hours, I soon came to depend on one of the charge nurses, Margaret Conlan, for breakfast and other snacks from the ward fridge. Cupboard love led later to the real thing—the liver brought us together, a sort of "love among the lobules," as it were—and we married a couple of years later.

Most of the patients were jaundiced and many had cirrhosis of the liver. The 50 beds on those two wards contained the largest concentration of people with liver disease in the U.K. and I felt privileged to be part of it, even though I was very uninformed. We had no Prof. Higgins here— or so I thought—so there were times when I felt like an old cabbage leaf.

Sherlock was in the throes of writing the first edition of her book on the liver, which became a classic, with many subsequent editions. I was fascinated by the research being done in the unit on patients who hovered on the brink of liver coma. The research team observed that when patients with stable chronic liver disease were asked to hold their arms straight out in front, some of their bodies and limbs had quite severe irregular jerky movements. This was called the "liver flap" and, in its more severe form, could be a sign of a pre-coma condition.

The research team thought that diet was somehow important in precipitating the slide into liver coma, but did not know how this happened or what aspect of diet was implicated. It was observed that coma was brought on by a hemorrhage into the oesophagus, which led to blood in the stomach and intestine—a fairly common state of affairs with chronic liver fibrosis (cirrhosis). This caused the team to suspect that the bleeding delivered a sudden high protein load to the individual's digestive system, so that, in effect, the individual digested his or her own blood protein. Thus, they speculated, the problem might be protein-related, though how this was so was not clear.

It did not seem likely that peptides—proteins that are broken down by the digestive enzymes of the gut—were the culprit. The researchers thought it more likely that the problem arose when the intestinal bacteria broke down the peptides and amino acids, producing excessive amounts of ammonia. A healthy liver can readily detoxicate gut-produced ammonia, but a chronically diseased liver has difficulty. Normally, a large volume of blood (containing the ammonia) flows through the portal vein from the intestine to the liver to be detoxified. However, fibrosis (scarring) inside

Figure 3.1 Pathway of ammonia absorption.

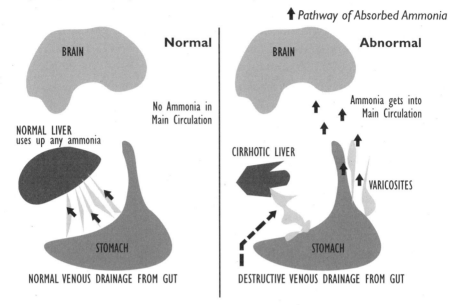

the liver obstructs the flow of the portal vein. As a result of this obstruction, the body creates bypass routes—esophageal varicose veins—that can carry a great deal of blood. The question was: Could these new bypasses provide a way for ammonia to get into the main blood stream without going through the liver (see Figure 3.1)? Free ammonia in the blood, normally absent, could affect the brain and cause the "liver flap" and induce pre-coma. This was the hypothesis.

The researchers hoped to find a way to prevent "liver flap" and the pre-coma condition, and hoped this might also help improve the health of patients with chronic cirrhosis of the liver. Because this condition can go on for years, the team reasoned that dietary protein restriction might lead to considerable improvement and might be important in longer-term management.

To test this hypothesis, they began a three-phase experiment:

1. First, a control group of patients with cirrhosis, but no bleeding, were given a high-protein diet to see if protein did, in fact, induce the flapping tremor of hepatic pre-coma. This was done on a number of patients and it proved to be a pre-coma precipitating factor.

2. A second group of patients with cirrhosis were then given an antibiotic aminoglycoside (Neomycin) and, after a few days, a

high-protein diet. The theory was that the antibiotic would kill the gut bacteria (resulting in what is called a partially sterile gut), thus preventing the bacterial breakdown of peptides and amino acids and the subsequent production of ammonia. They found that a high-protein load on a partially sterile gut did not precipitate the flapping tremor or hepatic pre-coma.

3. The third step was to determine whether the gut-produced ammonia spread through the body of a patient with chronic liver disease, or whether the liver could continue to clear it. The researchers compared these patients to normal subjects. Both were fed high-protein diets. Then blood was sampled from the arm veins and the hepatic vein—the vein leaving the liver—to see if there was increased levels of blood ammonium. For this it was necessary to place sampling tubes (venous catheters) from the large veins in the groin, through the heart and into the hepatic vein. They found that brain intoxication, as evidenced by confusion and an increase in tremors and flapping, was proportional to the rise of blood ammonia as shown, crudely, in Figure 3.1. There was no rise in blood ammonia in normal subjects.

Working all this out suggested a new way of treating and preventing early hepatic coma in chronic liver disease, especially when precipitated by protein in the diet (or blood in the stomach). I was proud to be on the unit while this research was being completed. The findings were widely acclaimed by those treating chronic liver disease, and remain relevant aspects of therapy to this day, but….Regrettably there is a *but*….and it has to do with values.

Some years later, in 1966, a Harvard anesthetist, Henry Beecher, in a now-famous classic paper[14] on medical ethics, identified and described in a general way a number of unethical reports in the literature that related to clinical research. Imagine my horror when a subsequent book published in 1991, *Strangers at the Bedside: A History of how Law and Bioethics transformed Medical Decision Making* by D.J. Rothwell,[15] gave all the details that were missing in Beecher's original article. This included one of Beecher's examples of unethical research concerning individuals with chronic liver disease who were studied during my period as house-officer at the Royal Post-Graduate Medical School, Hammersmith.[16] This revelation came as a considerable shock.

A LEGITIMATE INQUISITION OF
THE HOUSE-PHYSICIAN

What follows is a fictional account of questions an ethicist might have asked me about these experiments.

"Were you aware," the ethicist might ask, *"that patients in pre-hepatic coma could be protected by prior gut sterilization with the antibiotic Neomycin when challenged with protein feeding?"*

No, no one knew for sure—it was a hunch, I guess.

"Were you aware that the patients in the control group could readily be pushed into hepatic pre-coma by oral protein when not protected by oral sterilization of the gut?"

Yes, I soon became aware of this, but they could then readily be reversed from that pre-coma.

"But did they know what was happening, and had they given consent?"

Well, no! Not actually—but everything was done in their "best interests" if you use that term in a collective sense. [The classic cop-out.]

"But 'best interests' for a sick person must surely always be an individual thing; it is never to be construed as a collective interest, or the interest of the greatest number."

Yes, that is absolutely right, I suppose.

"What about the insertion of catheters into the hepatic veins? Was this a risky procedure in these sick people?"

Yes, it certainly was, as most people with chronic liver disease also have an increased tendency to bleed.

"And had they given fully-informed consent?"

No, they had not. I realize that, now!

"Were the research findings important?"

Yes. They established a method of management for early hepatic coma that is still used today.

"Does this justify the absence of consent?"

No, I regret to say, it does not.

"Another thing, was there scrutiny of each step in these experiments by a research ethics board?"

No. Such bodies had not been introduced anywhere in the 1953–1955 period. Research ethics depended on the researcher's integrity and patient trust.

"Do you think that relying on such factors was adequate?"

No, I guess not, in view of changing attitudes about these things and the fact that sometimes research subjects were injured.

"Was any person actually injured by these experiments?"

No, I have to say that I was not aware of any such accident during my nine-month watch on the Sherlock service.

"Did the conduct of the research, overall, seem to be unethical at the time?"

No, I have to say that it did not. And that is the scary part.

Ethical Dilemma

There were three breaches of research ethics in this clinical research from 1953 to 1955.

First, the patients who were given high-protein diets were not warned that it might put them into hepatic pre-coma (though we knew we could just stop the protein supplement if that happened).

Second, the patients were not warned that the protection against protein loads provided by the oral antibiotic posed some risk as well, and that it was not being done in their own immediate interest but in the pursuit of "generalizable knowledge"—a phrase that is used to describe the rationale for doing things that are not known to be in the direct interests of an individual patient.

Third, those selected for placement of tubes in their hepatic and other veins for ammonia measurements were not told that this carried risk and was not being done for their own immediate good, either.

All three aspects constituted serious breaches of the principle of informed consent.

This was my first involvement in ethically questionable clinical research, albeit as a junior on the team—one whose name did not appear on the publication—whose role, ironically enough, was to protect vulnerable patients from the exuberance and zeal of the clinical research team. The reader can understand my true consternation when I appreciated these shocking breaches of ethics, especially because I was a director of an ethics centre when I first came across this 1991 dénouement. It bothers me to this day that I was not alert enough to what was going on.

In retrospect, even in 1955, we should have been more aware and vigilant. The medical atrocities of World War II—done in the name of research—had been roundly condemned at the Nuremberg trial, yet we still had very little sensitivity regarding the ethical rights of research participants to comprehend the nature of clinical research. The sacrosanct nature of the doctor-patient relationship was such that patients trusted physicians not to do them harm. Further, they assumed that they, as patients, could only grasp the bare outline of a research project. One asked them to agree verbally for most things, including research. Only surgery required written consent. It is now obvious that the ends never justify the means. Fully informed and comprehended consent is a crucial aspect of treating others as moral equals and in showing them respect.

It was not until Beecher's paper was published in 1966 that the medical academic world began to wake up and realize it had to take medical ethics seriously. Fortuitously, this wake-up call came as clinical medical research was beginning a period of exponential growth, which lasts to this day. Although the Royal Post-Graduate Medical School at Hammersmith was the principal centre for clinical research in U.K., the main surge of research was in the U.S. After World War II, the U.S. Committee for Medical Research was converted into the National Institutes of Health (NIH), and the 500-bed Clinical Research Center was built at Bethesda, Maryland. NIH research funding grew from US$0.7 million in 1945, to US$35 million in 1955 to US$20 billion by 2001; a 20,000-fold increase over 56 years.

Despite the increase in funding and scope of research, investigators were still reluctant to accept the need for supervision of clinical research. In 1960, Prof. Lou Welt surveyed 80 U.S. medical schools and found only eight had documents for research ethics, and only 24 were in favour of having a Human Research Ethics Committee.[17]

Unfortunately, it required much more evidence of research harms before the medical world acknowledged that more supervision by third parties was necessary to protect the subjects whose experiences provided the raw data in this enormous search for new medical knowledge.

My postgraduate training continues

After my nine-month stint at Hammersmith Hospital, I did a six-month locum registrar position at Addenbroke's Hospital in Cambridge where I filled in for other internal medicine registrars who were away. I was then appointed registrar back at St. Bartholomew's Hospital, my training school, where I worked on the Geoffrey Bourne/Bodley Scott* firm, with Daryl Koch as my senior registrar. The main focus was general internal medicine and hematology.

Working in London, I was able to take advantage of various post-graduate sessions and courses. I attended the neurological sessions at

---

* Bodley, as he was known, was a descendent of a Bodley of Elizabethan 16th century times, after whom the Bodleian Library, Oxford, is named. Bodley was physician to the Queen's household, including butlers and so on. Later, Sir Bodley became the Queen's physician.

Queen's Square Hospital for Neurological Diseases, and took the MRCP exams. I even indulged in a modest social life, nearly all of it with beauteous companions (Margaret, Patricia, Dorothy, and Peggy), and lived with my mother, widowed now for 6 years, in her flat in Swiss Cottage. It was a satisfying time but I worried about the future.

I wanted to be involved in an academic specialty career in medicine (internal medicine) and this involved getting a senior registrarship at a teaching hospital, then waiting for one of the small number of consultancies to come available. In the mid-1950s, more than 100 applicants sought each registrarship of the type I cherished. It was depressing. So inbred were the London teaching hospitals that it was said that one got the job by marrying the right person, and that was it. With that in mind, I had found a way of taking out one of the daughters of Sir Bodley Scott. My dim recollection of that evening is that it was not a success, so I kept my eye on opportunities abroad and favoured the idea of Australia, my parents' homeland. I was also torn, though, because I did not want to leave my mother; I was the only single child, and her youngest.

A fateful decision, never to be regretted

About this time, my first chief and father figure in medicine, Prof. Christie, announced he was leaving Bart's to become a professor of medicine and physician-in-chief at the Royal Victoria Hospital (RVH) in Montreal. During his early research career in the 1930s he had spent time at McGill and in New York, and was well respected overseas. Before he left, I went to see him, thinking he could give me some assessment of my career chances in London, and perhaps a good reference.

Puffing away at a cigarette (he did not inhale, but nevertheless got through more than one pack a day), he said in his still obvious clipped Scottish accent, "Well now, Dossetor, you'll do well enough. I feel sure about that, but where that will be I don't know. I'll write the odd letter for you, for sure, but have you ever thought about going abroad?" I murmured vaguely about Australia. "Well, I don't know much about that, but if you would like to try a year or so in Canada, there is a teaching position at McGill that might suit you. It is an eight-month commitment, it's paid $200 a month—you are not married are you? My associate over there, one John Beck, told me it was open. How would you like that? Anyway, think about it and let me know tomorrow."

When I left him I felt a bit disappointed, but also kind of encouraged at the challenge. I called up Alex Aranof, a Canadian friend and gastroenterologist-in-training whom I had met at Hammersmith, and asked him about the reputation of the RVH and McGill University, and some other questions—including how far $200 a month would stretch in Montreal. I was still concerned about leaving my mother, but three of my siblings were living in the southern part of the England at that time, and I reasoned that Canada was a lot closer than Australia to the U.K., and my mother—a five-hour flight instead of a 24-hour journey. The fact that Margaret had moved to New York City a few months previously also factored into the equation.

The long and the short of it was that I was back in Prof. Christie's office the next day, saying I would like to try it. "Good, good," he said, "I'll let them know, but take it from me, its yours for the academic year, which starts in September—very soon, in fact." As a bit of an afterthought he added, "You are not coming as part of my team, you know that, eh? You are coming at the same time as me, but not with me. Okay, John? But it will be good to have you there. Come and see me the day after you arrive."

So, at the end of my first year of residency a decision to go to Canada as a Hosmer Teaching Fellow at McGill University Medical School was made within 24 hours, and I have never regretted it for a moment. In fact, it was a crucial turning point, and a wonderful opportunity for a 30-year-old with a spirit of adventure.

There is a tide in the affairs of men,
Which, taken at the flood, leads on to fortune;
Omitted, all the voyage of their life
Is bound in shallows and in miseries.
On such a full sea are we now afloat;
And we must take the current when it serves,
Or lose our ventures.

William Shakespeare (1564–1616)
Julius Caesar

4

The New World: Montreal, 1955–1961

As the SS *Seven Seas* steamed up the St. Lawrence River toward Montreal, the fall colouring of yellows and reds contrasted with the white spires of the Quebec parish churches, and the mood seemed tranquil and welcoming. Nonetheless, I felt some trepidation. I was committed to this venture for one year but I had no idea how it would turn out. At the back of my mind was the thought that well, it is only for a year. If worse came to worst, I could go back to England and renew my contacts in medicine there.

I arrived October 15 and spent my first night at the YMCA in the centre of the city. The next day I went up to the Royal Victoria Hospital (RVH) to meet briefly with Prof. Ronald Christie, my erstwhile chief at St. Bartholomew's Hospital in London, U.K., and Dr. John Beck, my new boss, and head of endocrinology and metabolism (He was supposed to meet me at the boat, but had failed to show up). Prof. Christie introduced me to the chief resident in medicine, Dr. Allan Knight, who later proved to be a great companion and life-long friend. Allan and his wife Yvonne made me feel very much at home and introduced me to *Hockey Night in Canada* and all the appropriate institutions of Canadian life. As chief resident, he conducted ward rounds on the public medical wards every evening and thus I was introduced to the ways of Canadian hospital medicine. The art of medicine is part science, which I expected to be the same in Canada as in U.K., part relational, or specific to each practitioner, and part culture, which is unique to each practice setting. It was this third component that I needed to learn.

A Hosmer teaching fellow at McGill

Being a teaching fellow allowed me to immerse myself in the medical culture. The medical students were friendly and seemed to appreciate my method of teaching physical signs in the clinical examination of patients. Much of this I had learned from Dr. Maurice Pappworth, whose medicine review sessions I had religiously attended while preparing for the Royal College of Physicians exam in London a year or so previous.

I was struck by how many of the medical class came from California. At that time, Californians comprised the largest state or provincial group of McGill's medical alumni, with the second largest coming from British Columbia. This was probably the result of family traditions and the delayed development of medical academia in the West; the University of British Columbia had graduated its first medical class just the year before.

The atmosphere at the RVH was definitely anglophone, and not very friendly towards Jewish people, either. There was a Jewish quota of about ten entrants per year at the medical school, which, I am glad to say, was soon to be abolished. I was not at all conscious of the French question in 1955; every Quebecer I met spoke English, even when I addressed them in what I hoped was French.

I paid $10 a week for a room on Shuter Street, which was within walking distance of the RVH. I ate at the local greasy spoon or the hospital cafeteria, and most of my spare change went to telephoning Margaret Conlan at the nurses residence at Mt. Sinai hospital in New York.

I served out my year as teaching fellow with great enjoyment and just as I was beginning to think about what I should do next, Prof. Christie offered me the position of chief resident in medicine for 1956–1957. It was an honour for me. He said, "You see, John, we both know the U.K. scene from the bedside viewpoint, but I don't know it over here. I need you to interpret it to me. We'll meet every morning at 9:00 and you can brief me on the previous 24 hours from the house-staff viewpoint, alright?"

"Right, Sir, and thank you very much!" I said.

And so I acted as a bridge for Prof. Christie to the clinical goings-on at the hospital, helping him to appreciate the differences between the U.K. and Canadian system. Generally, Canada's medical establishment was much less formally structured. In the U.K., the chiefs were looked upon as demi-gods and the rigid hierarchy made it exceedingly difficult for anyone, no matter how qualified, to become a consultant with the attendant

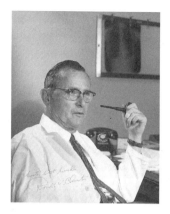
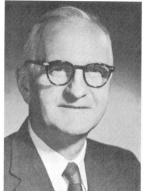

Prof. Ronald V. Christie (left), father figure and inspiration.
Dr. D. Ewan Cameron (right), who died with his reputation intact in 1967, has since been totally discredited for his research methods.

honour of teaching. In Canada, opportunities for advancement seemed to based more on *what* you knew, rather than *whom* you knew.

I was delighted to be so intimately involved in the operation of the RVH department of medicine, carrying out chief resident rounds on each day's admissions, arranging weekly medical grand rounds, and doing medical consultations in other parts of the hospital at night, with delegated authority from the attending staff, whom I relied upon for backup.

The ethical void in the sleep room

Among my nightly consultation duties was a passing involvement in an experiment that later became an infamous national and international example of medical research with seriously flawed ethics. It has more recently become notorious through a CBC television documentary and the prize-winning book, *In the Sleep Room*.[18]

Dr. Ewan Cameron, head of psychiatry in the RVH's Allen Memorial Institute wing was seen as a great innovator who might—just might—blow open a whole new way of mind management for psychiatric disorders that would leave the Freudian psychoanalysts way behind. The idea was to use physical mind-management techniques to first deconstruct the mind and sponge out all previous behaviour patterns, then second, to re-implant ideas derived from listening to tapes while asleep—so-called psychic driving. If successful, this technique would allow patients to preclude tedious and expensive one-on-one psychoanalysis. Cameron was testing several techniques for depatterning the mind: multiple electroconvulsive therapies (ECTs); hallucinogen lysergic acid (LSD) drug therapy; days of drug-induced sleep; and/or long periods of insulin-induced very low blood sugar (insulin stupor).

As head of the psychiatry department and past-president of the American Psychiatric Association (1952–1953), Cameron's psychiatric colleagues seemed to lap up his theory and hold him in great esteem, even awe. He was considered an intellectual powerhouse who could do not wrong; his reputation, locally, nationally and internationally was Olympian. Perhaps as a result, Cameron had medical hubris to an extreme degree. He demanded unconditional trust from those he elected to treat and those who were members of his team. His patients loved him and thought the man was an inspiration. I am sure they felt they could trust him implicitly—indeed, he engendered trust. I am also sure he thought he was helping them, but that is not good enough, not by a very long way.

It later turned out that the U.S. Central Intelligence Agency (CIA) was supporting the research through a philanthropic front organization, the Society for Investigation of Human Ecology, later renamed the Human Ecology Fund (an euphemism, if ever there was one). The CIA was interested in mind-bending, brainwashing and similar techniques, and gladly funded the Canadian psychiatrist at McGill who was prepared to do research for them.

Part of my job as the RVH's chief medical resident was to respond to consultation calls at night at the Allen Memorial Institute. Of course, I did not know the full nature of the protocol. All I knew was that the patient was under drug-induced sleep therapy or controlled insulin coma, or that the night nurses were worried about some after-effect or other of the heavy ECT.

Cameron rode roughshod over all concepts of patients' rights and informed consent as well as his professional responsibility to the Hippocratic axiom *primum non nocere* (first, do no harm). Regrettably, no one seemed to realize how useless and dangerous this approach was, and certainly no one said anything. There was an assumption that the treatment had been explained to the patients and that they had consented, but there was no written evidence of this. There must have been some patients who had early benefits (as Dr. Peter Roper strongly contended), otherwise there would have been an immediate outcry. But it is the adverse long-term effects that amply show how wrongly conceived was the whole of this research, both scientifically and from the standard of research ethics.

Though this is an extreme case, its underpinnings were not unusual at the time. Along with most of my colleagues, I was deficient in our awareness of the rules of research, despite the fact that I was hoping, and

Ethical Dilemma

Cameron had no research plan or protocol that others could review (at that time, there were no research ethics boards). There was no formal consent process for research subjects, no valid method of result assessment, no outside review of a totally unproved methodology, and scant attention to privacy or confidentiality. This research was done on whim and assessed on a whim using non-scientific methodology. Even if some of the patients may have benefited, it was still disgraceful. It was unethical in just about every meaning of that phrase. "Trust me—I know what's good for you," was the paternalistic philosophy under which this research was conducted.

On the nights when I saw patients at the institute, I was, in fact, an accomplice to unethical research. It is scary to recognize, yet again, one's lack of sensitivity to patients' rights, and the obligation to respect their dignity and autonomy. It underscores the need to protect humans in research from irresponsible clinical investigators. Pappworth, who helped me prepare for my U.K. exams, wrote in his 1967 book: "No physician is justified in placing science or the public welfare first and his obligation to the individual who is his patient second. No doctor, however great his capacity or original his ideas has the right to choose martyrs for science or for the general good."[19] I could not agree more.

How much harm resulted from this psychiatric experimentation—albeit carried out supposedly in the "patient's best interest"? Several aspects allow one to conclude that it caused serious harm. Patients claimed that they lost memory for long periods of time before and subsequent to intense depatterning. These patients far outnumber those for whom the treatment was beneficial. In support of this conclusion was the 20-year struggle Cameron's patients fought before they received compensation from the Allen Memorial Institute and the RVH, as well as his sources of research funding (the CIA and, later, the Canadian government).

In the Sleep Room documents the long struggle of David Orlikow, then a Member of Parliament from Winnipeg, on behalf of his wife, Val, and the equally valiant efforts of lawyers J.L. Rauh and his partner Jim Turner (both based in Washington). There were no court judgements attributing guilt, but there were eventual settlements. In 1981 the RVH settled out of court with the Orlikows for approximately $50,000. In the U.S., the CIA also settled out of court for US$750,000 with six plaintiffs, but with no admission of liability. Finally, in 1992, the Canadian government passed the AMI-Depatterned Persons Assistance Order, which authorized payments of $100,000, *ex gratia*, to any Canadian resident who could prove that he or she had been subjected to Cameron's experiments in brainwashing, after each signed a waiver promising no further court action. Seventy-seven people received the payment.[20] These cases are tragic. For example, AMI records show that between May 1 and September 12, 1963, Linda Macdonald of Vancouver underwent more than 100 electroshock treatments and 86 days of drugged sleep with intensive psychic driving. She emerged completely disorientated, and incontinent.[21]

expecting, to develop a career in clinical research. This career choice had gradually emerged over a long period. It began when I worked with Dame Sherlock's unit, and grew under Prof. Christie back at Bart's. I wanted to specialize in internal medicine, but was hooked on clinical research. I had an overwhelming desire to investigate things that would improve people's life in a direct way. I also felt exceedingly fortunate to participate in what was really a new type of research. Previously, research had been mostly concerned with accurate descriptions of disease as it developed—the so-called natural history of disease—or experiments in the laboratory, probably with animals. There were not enough tools to do prospective clinical trials (a study that starts with the present condition of a population of individuals and follows them into the future). Investigative clinical research, or medical research at the bedside, really started in the 1950s and 1960s, during what I have termed the third epoch (see Appendix 1). This new type of research meant that patients would be used as subjects, making my lack of knowledge about medical ethics potentially even more dangerous.

BEYOND THE HIPPOCRATIC OATH

An unusual case

My year as chief medical resident had some notable moments, too. I was doing rounds one evening on the public ward and with great alarm thought a newly-admitted, extremely overweight women was dead. She was lying there, passive, massive, not breathing and blue in the face. She had been admitted with possible Cushing's syndrome (an adrenal or pituitary hyperfunction that causes an excess secretion of corticosteroids, especially hydocortisone). Such patients are bluish and obese, but not like this one. We ran across the ward to her bedside, pulled the screens around her bed, and pounced on her. She opened her eyes and said "What are you boys up to?" or words to that effect. Quickly she became pink again. Cushing's syndrome patients would not pink up like that.

On studying her closely, we realized that her primary problem was a weak drive to breathe adequately, and it came to mind that a similar hypo-ventilation condition had been recently described and associated with excessive obesity—for the first time, I believe—in the *American Journal of Medicine*.[22] In this condition, a patient's drive to breathe becomes depressed when drowsy and he or she behaves exactly as this woman behaved. It is sometimes referred to as Pickwickian fat boy syndrome. We later proved this to be the diagnosis, and she was one of the patients whom I asked to participate as a subject for the clinical part of the Royal College Fellowship in Internal Medicine examination being held in Montreal that year. This woman agreed and was presented as the long case to a candidate from the cardiology service at The Cleveland Clinic, who was a Canadian trainee there. He got the diagnosis right away.

The problem is that the chief examiner, a senior physician at the RVH, had never heard of this admittedly very rare condition. I guess he was behind in his reading of the *American Journal of Medicine*. He determined that the differential diagnosis should include Cushing's disease, and some other entities. The hotshot candidate from The Cleveland Clinic said, "No, Sir, there is nothing else it can be, when someone pinks up like that." His confidence certainly did not bring him luck. An enraged and disappointed man returned to Cleveland from Montreal that night. I felt outraged as well.

This reminds me of an adage from my excellent instructor, Pappworth: When dealing with examiners of the Royal College (in his case he was referring to the Royal College of Physicians in London, U.K., but the advice still stands), it is always better to be an anencephalic than a smart Alec. I have since passed that advice to many smart candidates for clinical exams, and I believe it has served them well.

Ethical Dilemma

This brings up a delicate dilemma of professional ethics. To what extent should one trust the knowledge of senior medical examiners in oral examinations? Their knowledge is sometimes quite limited on certain points—even though they are considered reliable and well-informed overall. The possibility of injustice to candidates is guarded against, to some extent, by examiners working in pairs, so that one can correct (usually at a later moment) a possible error or injustice on the part of the other. But this is not always possible during a bedside examination.

The system has other safeguards as well. Examiners are appointed by their senior peers, rotate off the examiners' roster after a few years, are not allowed to examine candidates they have helped train, and must declare any conflict of interest in favour or disfavour of each candidate they see.

The best one can say, I think, is that the system, with its weaknesses, is the same for each candidates, but that does little to help those who are subjected to unfair prejudice or ignorance on the part of their oral examiners. Moreover, as a rule, there is no appeal process and a failed candidate is going to think twice before writing to the chief examiner about a perceived possible injustice.

The importance of communication

The responsibilities of a senior resident are many, but most especially it is the resident's duty to look after people with difficult medical problems that are not yet adequately understood and are undergoing investigation. He or she is also responsible for the quality of the care received by ward patients from medical staff, especially the other residents, in association with nursing staff and others. The lesson I carried away from this 12-month experience is that nearly everything that goes wrong in the smooth running of a large institution—including unethical situations—occurs because of poor interpersonal communication, often resulting from poor interpersonal relationships.

Many excuses are used to avoid good honest direct personal communication, and some of these are legitimate, no doubt. But the fact remains that, in the absence of deliberately planned good communications (written and otherwise), all sorts of problems arise, suppurate and eventually burst. Only some of these poor communications are intended with malice; more often they are due to laziness, false expediency, too many commitments, or insensitivity to the crucial role of good relationships in our struggle to provide ethical health care.

Ethical Dilemma

Shift-work presents a poignant example of how inadequate staff relationships and communications can lead to substantial, indeed life-threatening, problems. In the daily grind of being on duty from 7:00 a.m. to 5:00 p.m. then handing over to another resident for the night, it is too easy to overlook the simple fact that one is handing over the care of sick, vulnerable people. It is totally different, in ethical terms, from leaving the factory floor and letting the night shift take over. How, then, should one deal with this periodic shifting of professional responsibility? The answer lies in the adequacy of the verbal hand-over, in making oneself available even when off duty to answer special aspects of an individual's care, and in the written communication one leaves in the patient record, which states what might be expected in that person's case. Thus, in this sense, the responsibility remains with each participating physician, even when off duty.

Another safeguard is to have staggered professional responsibility, with overlapping coverage, such as that which occurs when a senior member of staff hands over care to a resident by means of a ward round and then goes back to his or her office. One should also ensure that the nursing staff's shift changes do not occur at the same time as the resident physicians' so that there is an overlap in professional care.

The working life of residents has improved over the years, but what has not changed is this ongoing responsibility for the care of people in a hospital. That can never be completely shed as one leaves the ward to go home. And this will always be so, as I see it, no matter how good the working conditions become.

Later, I will return to this aspect of professionalism, as distinct from those occupations that do not deal with vulnerable humanity, when we consider how best to hand over responsibility of care:

- in a kidney dialysis unit where people with chronic renal failure are being treated day in and day out by a changing team of professionals and
- on an intensive care unit (ICU) where *senior* medial staff rotations may be no longer than a week at a time and yet patients may be in the unit for weeks.

There are strong ethical implications for health professionals in these situations and they are not diminished—indeed, they may be glossed over—by the efficiency with which rosters are made out and circulated to others (nurses, switchboard operators, other colleagues, and the like).

A call to sack the chief medical resident—me!

As for the difficult medical problems during this time, one stands out from the rest. A pregnant woman bearing her first child had serious chronic rheumatic heart disease. She went into acute heart failure and had to be admitted to obstetrics late one Saturday afternoon as an emergency with premature delivery. Her heart was enlarged, her lungs were congested, her pulse was thready, her cardiac rhythm was rapid and irregular and her blood pressure was low. As the chief medical resident, I was called to see her and advise on treatment. I examined her and contacted the attending cardiologist on call. She was clearly gravely ill. We discussed various possibilities and decided on slow digitalization, partly because we did not know (she only spoke Greek) how much digitalis she might have been given by others in the immediate past. The cardiogram was abnormal, but did not exclude the possibility of the digitalis having a beneficial effect. We gave her oxygen, improved her position in bed, and, as a temporary measure, administered a medical venesection (using a cuff above venous pressure to cause blood to pool in the periphery) while watching vital signs very carefully. We were planning a true venesection—removal of one litre of blood.

The cardiologist said he would be there in an hour. This was before the days of cardiac resuscitation teams and cardiac intensive care units. Before the cardiologist arrived, she died quite suddenly. Why? Rhythm change into ventricular fibrillation? Insufficient digitalization? Pulmonary embolus? We were all shocked, but the obstetrical chief-of-service erupted with rage. He was convinced that the fault was mine. He ranted at me and at the cardiologist and at the department of medicine. He also wrote a furious letter to Prof. Christie, saying that I was incompetent and had allowed a patient of his to die. He demanded that I be sacked!

I was called to Christie's office at 9:00 the next morning. I did not know what to expect. I did not feel I had been as effective as I should have been, for some reason, but at the same time, I did not think that I should carry the blame for her death, though I was very distraught over it. Christie peered at me and said: "The chief of obstetrics is demanding that you be sacked. What have you got to say about it?" His tone, though solemn, was not angry. I went into an explanation, but it turned out that he had already talked at length to the cardiologist.

"John," he said, "if I didn't know that you could handle catastrophes like this, I would not have appointed you. Now that we have had this experience, you will be a better physician because of it. It is fortunate that everyone corroborates what you did, and would have done essentially the same. It is fortunate, also, that I know [the obstetric chief] from way back when. He is known to be a bully. Go back to your work. You did just

Ethical Dilemma

The ethics issues here are complex and I have never felt able to resolve them. Without a full factual investigation—which was not carried out because the obstetrical chief's letter immediately raised the level of the problem to its maximum by peremptorily demanding severe disciplinary action—it is not possible to judge whether there was negligence, ignorance, or both, on my part, or whether others simply needed to accept the inevitable. Today, an intensive resuscitation team with capability to intubate and artificially ventilate might have saved her life, and possibly that of her child. Such teams were not introduced until the early 1960s. But the unfortunate fact remains that grave things happen to those who are gravely ill. *Such is the great uncertainty of the practice of medical care.*

Still, there were ethical breeches in this case. An autopsy should have been done, but was not. That was a serious omission. The trust between consulting services was breached by the severity of the accusation, and that is not in the patient's best interest—ever. My chief's defence of me testified to the strength and value of our relationship, but did not answer the question of negligence either way. The one positive outcome was that my sensitivity to ethical issues in health care increased sharply.

fine even though it was a medical disaster. They happen, you now know. Forget about his inappropriate rage. I will write him to say that I am pleased to affirm you as my chief resident!"

I was greatly relieved. So, for the third time in my career, Christie had given me courage and shown thoughtful insight.

A nephrologist is born

During my year as chief resident, I embarked on another life-changing experience when Margaret and I married on February 9, 1957, in New York City, then moved back as a couple, to Montreal. Our first child, Frances, was born late that year; twins, John and Clare, followed in 1959; and Moira was born in 1963.

Back on the work front, some months after the end of the medical residency in 1957, I sat the examinations for the Fellowship of the Royal College of Physicians of Canada with specialization in internal medicine. One memento of the occasion is the $100 cheque I sent for my entry fee, which was returned by the Registrar marked I.S.F. (insufficient funds). I guess they tried to cash it towards the end of the month. They should have known better. I count myself as likely to be the only physician who sent the Royal College a cheque that bounced!

With my exam out of the way, I concentrated on developing a specialty within the field of internal medicine. I had previously had opportunities to specialize in heart disease (cardiology at the U.K. National Heart Hospital) and liver disease (hepatology, at the Royal Post-Graduate Medical School in London), and was considering the latter. Prof. Christie said they would quite like to keep me around RVH and asked what I wanted to do next. I said, somewhat diffidently, "Well, I don't really know. I had wondered about liver disease as a specialty."

"Well," he said, "you know, John, I am not sure that we really need someone to build in that area, but I have been speaking with John Beck and we wondered if you would care to become a nephrologist and build up the kidney side of our work here—we don't have anyone in that area now that Michael Kaye has moved to the Montreal General."

I stood silent before him, thinking it over, and the chief continued. "We could arrange for you to go and learn kidney biopsy with Robert Kark, C.L. Pirani and Victor Pollak in Chicago, at the Presbyterian Hospital there. We know Kark because he used to be here at the Vic, years ago. After you have learned how to do kidney biopsies, you can come back here and be a nephrologist. And we have some funds to send you there for a week or so. How does that prospect seem to you?"

I concurred; it seemed too good an invitation to turn down.

I went to Chicago and back by bus—the grant was not a very large one—but I was very hospitably treated. I learned how to do the kidney biopsies and returned to Montreal as the nephrologist at the RVH. That is all it took in those days: the word from the chief, and the ability to bring back a new gimmick! Mind you, there was no formal training for nephrology in 1958, no certification. I suppose I was one of three or so such people in all of Canada at the time. (By 1970 there were 300 nephrologists, and by 1999 about 600.) I have never regretted, for a moment, launching myself on that particular "tide in the affairs of men"; so many good things flowed from that decision.

A research fellowship and supervised consultations

The next year, 1957–1958, was eventful indeed; in retrospect it was the year that defined my future in medicine. On the advice of Beck and Prof. Christie, I applied for and got a Canadian Life Insurance Co. research fellowship to work in Beck's Division of Endocrinology and Metabolism. My colleague, Dr. Robert O. Morgen, and I constituted an "electrolyte, water and kidney" subdivision. I had become very interested in problems associated with salt and water, the acidity of the blood (acidosis), and the ensuing renal and adrenal pathophysiology.

New technologies had increased the potential for learning more about the body's water and electrolyte metabolism. These included:

- the flame photometer, which allowed rapid assays of sodium and potassium on serum, urine and other fluids;
- the osmometer, which measures osmotic force (positive and negative ions). We used the depression of small amounts of urine or serum's freezing point as a means of assaying overall solute content (the measurement of osmolarity gives the total content of molecules in a solution, regardless of ionic charge); and,
- the Astrup apparatus, which allowed us to measure the partial pressures of gases in anerobic blood (blood collected without exposure to air). With this technology we could rapidly measure blood acidity (or its pH) and the partial pressure of dissolved carbon dioxide; we could use this

information to calculate the plasma bicarbonate concentration in very small samples of blood.

These technologies, readily applied at the bedside, opened up a whole new field of clinical investigation and management of acid-base disorders and body electrolyte control. I was so fascinated by this field that I enrolled myself in a doctorate program in experimental medicine at McGill University to study the diurnal rhythm (24-hour rhythm) of electrolyte secretion and kidney function. The kidney normally excretes more during the day and less at night, which can be bothersome to people on shift work, who find their sleep interrupted by the urge to urinate, but after several months this pattern can change. I studied people on shift work, as well as patients at the in the Montreal Neurological Hospital who were in an unconscious coma (who retained the normal diurnal rhythm) and a persistent vegetative state (who did not).

My turn as a research subject

In the summer of 1957, I also enrolled myself as a research subject in an endocrinology experiment being conducted by a research fellow from Alberta, Dr. Lionel E. McLeod. I mention this episode not only for its ethical implications, but also because it provided me with first-hand experience of dehydration, which I subsequently drew upon during ethics consultations concerning end-of-life issues, where voluntary dehydration is discussed as one simple alternative to assisting another's suicide or getting involved in euthanasia.

The adrenal corticosteroid laboratory at McGill was world-class, and the team of Drs. Beck, J.S.L. Browne and Eleanor Venning were forerunners in the measurement of various adrenal steroids. In 1956, their main interest was in a new hormone, aldosterone, which acted on the kidney, causing it to retain sodium and promote potassium excretion. They were able to assay for aldosterone in blood and urine and were studying the effect of various physiological stresses on its excretion. McLeod's experiment involved measuring aldosterone under the stress of severe dehydration.

The experimental diet consisted of four identical meals a day, each as dry as possible. I had no free fluid in the form of water, tea or coffee, and the food itself was dry. My urine was collected every six hours. I was on my honour not to drink from the shower or the faucet. In fact, I experienced little difficulty in sticking to that promise. I can attest to the claim that thirst does not last. By the second day, I was aware of having a dry mouth, and was a bit light-headed, but the thirst had gone. In fact, even on the first day, I did not have what could be called a raging thirst, providing the mucous membranes of my mouth were moistened periodically.

As the week wore on, I found I was lethargic by day but my mind was alert—observers told me I seemed somewhat euphoric—and I had vivid, emotionally charged dreams at night. As I recall, I was in a sort of hallucinatory state. I mention this because I have since verified that those who wish to end their own lives by refusing food and fluid also experience a sort of trance-like state as they become progressively dehydrated.

At the end of the seven days, I had lost 6.4 kilograms (14 pounds) and did not feel too bad—just weak. I was allowed to rehydrate myself at my own speed, and I remember sitting in the hospital bed, the side table swung across in front of me, with my arms around several two-litre jugs of cold water. I put those 6.4 kilograms back on in about 30 minutes by simply drinking water, and then felt quite ill with a headache, a sort of fullness of the head. I was annoyed with McLeod for not warning me about this possibility, and not waiting to see me right through to the end of the experiment. Obviously he did not anticipate that I might rehydrate myself too quickly, and so go through a phase of what I am sure was cerebral edema, a mild swelling of the brain. Ethically speaking, I should have been warned and monitored. However, this ill effect only lasted a few hours, and I was fine when I went home that evening.

The results of this experiment, along with other clinical studies, formed part of the material for McLeod's master of science thesis,[*] and a couple of subsequent publications.

A career-making experience: The first kidney transplant in the Commonwealth

Concurrent with my research, I was a junior consulting physician, one of two nephrologists in a recently formed renal service. Dr. Robert O. Morgen (later at Baylor University in Houston, Texas) was the other. We were proud of the emergence of this new service, inspired by a questionable capacity for treating acute renal failure by hemodialysis, a conceit in manipulating electrolyte imbalance, and proven dexterity in wielding the renal biopsy needle.

---

[*] McLeod LE. Experiences in the measurement of various body fluid compartments. Presented to the Faculty of Graduate Studies and Research for the Degree of Master of Science, McGill University, Montreal, July 1957.

One holiday Monday, March 31, 1958, when I was on call as a metabolism and kidney consultant while Morgen enjoyed some spring skiing, Moira, a 15-year-old high-schooler, was admitted to the Montreal Neurological Institute (now hospital). She had severe epileptiform seizures and was pre-comatose with a high blood pressure. The metabolism and endocrinology service was asked to see her because of her high blood pressure and high serum potassium. It soon became apparent that she was in renal failure. An open renal biopsy confirmed a diagnosis of chronic pyelonephritis (inflammation of the kidney and its pelvis). A longstanding chronic infection had apparently left her with only about five per cent kidney function. The outlook was grim: she had six months, a year at most, to live. Little did I realize that this particular consultation would change my whole professional career.

Dr. Hélène Désjardins, the admitting resident at the Neurological Institute who had taken Moira's history from her mother, noted that the young woman had an identical twin sister and suggested than an identical-twin transplant might be a possibility. Normally the body will graft only onto itself; for example, fingers can be reattached, but the body rejects any alien material (someone else's finger, or kidney). Given the limits of medical therapy in 1958, Moira's body would have destroyed the kidney from anyone else save her identical twin.

At that time, no one in Canada had seriously addressed the question of renal transplantation. Worldwide, there had been only five instances of successful identical-twin transplants, all at the Peter Bent Brigham Hospital in Boston, which had been reported a year or so earlier.[23]

Dialysis, too, was in its infancy and because it was always carried out late in the course of renal failure, many patients died. Moira was stuporous—that is, her response to any stimulation was greatly diminished—but we wanted to avoid the risk of dialysis, which was, at that time, considered a measure of last resort. This is hard to believe nowadays, when it would be considered negligent not to dialyse her back to full consciousness and vigour using the artificial kidney before deciding on any other course of action. But this was 1958, so we instituted a meticulous control of fluids, electrolytes and protein, and hoped that we would not be pushed by progress in her renal failure into having to do a dialysis.

We explored the situation during the next few days, and I offered to send Moira to Boston for the transplant with Nola, her sister, as a potential kidney donor. They would accept her, but the expense would not be

Ethical Dilemma

Should live genetically-related kidney donors be accepted? Should physicians be operating on completely healthy people, for any purpose whatsoever? What about the axiom: *primum non nocere?*

There's also the question of determining the actual willingness of the donor. In a later case, a young man donated a kidney to his brother, but the graft had a vascular complication and failed and had to be removed within two weeks. As he left the hospital, he said to me, "Well, Doc, I guess the family will be satisfied with me, now, anyways." This was the first intimation that the family had pressured him to donate a kidney, and that there was some reluctance on his part.

Generally, it was deemed that the related adult kidney donor had a sufficiently strong compassionate motive for giving one kidney, and the practice became widespread once it became increasingly clear that the loss of one kidney did not lead to hypertension or other problems later in life. Of course, it took 20 to 30 years to fully realize this, but the early encouraging, and measurable, aspect was that the function of the remaining kidney rapidly increased towards achieving the functional capacity of two. We had first shown this rapid gain in function of a single kidney in our studies on the recipient of the identical-twin kidney transplant in 1958, Moira.

covered. We offered to help raise the money, but the twins were part of a closely-knit family of five daughters and one son, and their mother, strongly supported by the rest of the family, resolved to have her daughter stay at the RVH in Montreal. We carefully explained what we intended to do—but also that we had never done such a procedure before. They nonetheless agreed.

As the renal physician, supported by Beck and Morgen, my role was to orchestrate the whole affair from a medical planning viewpoint, with the help of two house-officers and a nursing team, and support from hospital administration.

Preparations for this first transplantation in any of the Commonwealth countries were prodigious, even though there was no need for clinical immunosupression (a term whose time was yet to come). During the

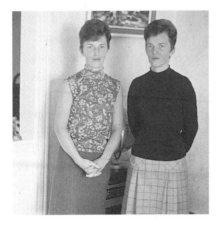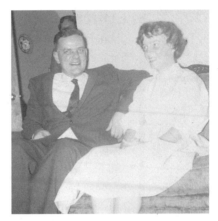

The Johnson twins (left), post-operatively (Nola on the left, Moira on the right). Moira Johnson, post-transplant, with one of her attending physicians (right). She was the first kidney transplant recipient in the Commonwealth and the sixth in the world.

workup we had to establish, as far as possible, that the twins were indeed biologically identical (born from the same egg). At the time DNA testing did not exist; instead, we used a series of observations and analyses to push the statistical odds that the young women were identical twins. Geneticists at McGill examined physical characteristics, including the colour and texture of hair and iris, ear and tooth shape, finger and toe prints, and blood type. In addition, we tested Nola to ensure that her kidney was functioning normally and we then had to show that exchanged skin grafts would not be rejected. A piece of skin from each was grafted to the other to see if the body could be fooled. It was.

Finally, we had to arrange for the actual transplantation, including preplanning for as complete a balance of fluid and salt changes as was possible. But we were also prepared to take on the risks of dialysis if these balances were insufficient to maintain some stability.

Before the transplantation, a family court judge had to grant the parents the right to give permission for nephrectomy—considered "a mutilation procedure"—on the healthy twin, who was a minor and could not give valid consent. I even had an unusual discussion with the RCMP because I had loosely said in a press interview that the twin sisters "even had identical fingerprints!" "Our information, doctor," said the RCMP officer, "is that even identical twins have distinctive sets of fingerprints." I am sure he was right!

On the appointed day, May 25, 1958, all went remarkably smoothly. The surgeons had planned their different procedures, but there was one strange moment. When implanting the donated kidney into Moira, the vascular surgeon, Dr. Joe C. Luke, joined the blood vessels meticulously, and then said, just before he stood back to leave the field for Dr. Ken MacKinnon, the urologist-in-chief, "We must clear up the field for Ken. He won't want these odd tags lying around, will he?" With that, he trimmed off some redundant tissue but also, to everyone's horror, the donor ureter. It was planned to use that structure to connect the donated kidney to Moira's bladder! A palpable shock shuddered through the operating room! We all thought that the donor's ureter was vital to success. But MacKinnon, with admirable *sang-froid*, seeing what had been done, immediately said, "We'll use Moira's old ureter. That has its natural junction with the bladder, and I'll just sew the ends together higher up." I, as a spectator in the OR, experienced an incredible feeling of relief.

Despite the lack of experience in performing this particular procedure, the surgery went very well. At that time, it was thought that a kidney could not survive more than 90 minutes without its blood supply. Nola's donated kidney was cut off from blood supply for only 58 minutes—just three over the record set in Boston. The operation took three more hours to complete. Even before the ureter was attached, the newly-placed kidney from Nola was bulging with fresh urine, and seeking a way out. On completion, there was an immediate brisk flow (or diuresis) and it was wonderful to see that golden liquid evidence of renewed life expectation.

In the next few days, while we frantically balanced intakes and outputs of fluid, sodium, potassium, magnesium, chloride, phosphate and bicarbonate, Moira bounded back to exuberant life. Maintaining precise fluid balance was a bit tricky because she had been very deeply in renal failure, and all those retained materials caused a fast urine flow. Eleven litres of urine were excreted in the first day, carrying out a lot of salts (normal urine output is between 800 mL and 1.6 litres per day).[24,25] Three nurses were assigned to the case, which was clearly excessive, but reflects the uncertainty of the management team. Nola was back home within ten days; Moira stayed four weeks. The greatest risk was infection, thus her room was kept as sterile as an OR. Her nurses had to change clothes every time they entered the room and Moira was not allowed books, radio, flowers or gifts. Instead, she read her charts.

The success of this whole operation was a great thrill to all those involved. The ethical issues were not great. Obviously, we had to have consent from both participants, and both parents. Looking back, it all seems quite unexciting from a medical point of view, but at the time it seemed to be epoch-making.

Moira lived another 29 years, just past her 40th birthday, and finally succumbed to cancer in 1987 (although her kidney failed in 1974, and she was on dialysis until her death). Nola still lives in Ottawa and we visit from time to time. My wife and I named our fourth child in honour of Moira.

So it was that consultation on that Monday afternoon of a long weekend that determined my whole future career. Kidneys? Yes. Kidney transplantation? Maybe. But cardiology or liver disease? No way, José!

Research fellow in New York

It would take another year to finish up my doctoral thesis and, since I had already spent two years on the Canadian Life Insurance Fellowship, I needed another source of funding. I also needed to do some experiments on animals. McGill did not have a primate animal lab, so I looked south of the border. Thus, I spent a year (1960–1961) as a U.S. Public Health Service Post-Doctoral Fellow, working next to Bellevue Hospital at New York University with Dr. Larry Wesson in the penumbra of the greatest renal physiologist of the century, Dr. Homer S. Smith, who had just retired but still came into the lab at regular intervals. My studies concerned the patterns of electrolyte excretion in the urine of dogs and a rhesus monkey. My quest was to understand the connection between the brain and the circadian rhythms of urinary excretion (diurnal fluctuations), and of kidney function as measured by renal physiological parameters. I spent many long hours studying the monkey, including nights sleeping on a camp cot in the lab during the experiments. The thought did occur to me, as I lay there, that my rhesus friend probably thought he was doing research on me and not the reverse. I must say there were moments when he may have been philosophically right in thinking so, especially because Margaret, with three toddlers—three-year-old Frances and two-year-old twins, John and Clare—lodged in a house on Staten Island, was in need of all the help I could give.

This work on diurnal changes in renal function and urine composition was completed, written up, submitted and defended—involving two trips from New York to Montreal—in time for the summer convocation at McGill in 1961.[*] My tentative conclusion was that the 24-hour rhythm was under control of the hypothalamus. It led to several subsequent publications.

Indecision

At this point, I was very clear that I wanted to pursue clinical research, not animal research or basic science, and that it should be in kidney disease, and possibly kidney transplantation, if that area was also going to develop (though nobody knew for sure). I explored various options in the U.S., keeping an offer to go back to McGill in my back pocket. The immediate options were the Mayo Clinic in Rochester, Minnesota, and the university medical schools at Houston, Texas, and Chapel Hill, North Carolina. The offer at the Mayo Clinic resulted from a contact with my long-time Oxford and Hammersmith friend, Dr. Bill Summerskill, who had gone there as a liver specialist and gastroenterologist. But it was made clear to me, much as I was impressed by the Mayo Clinic and its physicians, that it was not a place for those who really wanted time in the lab or to make clinical research a main objective.

Nor did I feel comfortable at the other two places. At Chapel Hill, renal patients were segregated into black and white wards, with corresponding differences in comfort and probably standards of care, though I had no evidence of the latter suspicion. There were slightly different drawbacks at Houston. They were really looking for a renal physician to take care of the post-operative renal problems that attended Dr. Michael DeBakey's very active and renowned cardiology surgery service. I did not want that. (Among DeBakey's many later accomplishments was being part of the team that did open-heart surgery on President Yeltsin in Moscow in the mid-1990s, when DeBakey was about 80 years old.) Also, at Houston, dialysis machines were not available—at that time, I stress—for African Americans with acute renal failure. I found these limitations to be more than I could feel comfortable with.

In any event, as McGill had good things to offer, we elected to go back to Canada and we have never regretted that decision.

* Dossetor JB. Studies of diurnal electrolyte excretion. Thesis submitted to the Faculty of Graduate Studies and Research in partial fulfillment of the requirements for the degree of Doctor of Philosophy, April 1961.

Returning to Canada

In 1961, the McGill Faculty of Medicine had a proud record—and still has—with an enviable reputation for academic medicine and research. Among the names I recall are Drs. Wilder Penfield, William Cone and Francis McNaughton in neurology and neurosurgery; endocrinologists John L.S. Brown and Eleanor Venning, who were instrumental in working out the hormone cycles that control menstruation and the changes that occur in pregnancy; Dr. Jonathan Meakins and Prof. Christie in pulmonary disease; Dr. Ewan Cameron in psychiatry (though his repute was soon to plunge into ignominy); Lyman Duff in pathology; and David Thomson in biochemistry. Physiology soon attracted Dr. Arnold Bergen from Cambridge as the head of the university department. The school and faculty received what seemed to be a disproportionate percentage of Medical Research Council funding and believed itself, through the usual processes of academic hubris, to be a cut above other medical schools in Canada.

I was given a very warm welcome back to the RVH, and now had the title of Director of Urological Research (with Ken MacKinnon, the head of urology) and Director of the Renal Failure Service.

II. Nephrology

For there are two modes of acquiring knowledge, namely, by reasoning and experience. *Reasoning* draws a conclusion and makes us grant the conclusion, but does not make the conclusion certain, nor does it remove doubt so that the mind may rest on the intuition of truth, unless the mind discovers it by the path of *experience*....

Roger Bacon, philosopher, 1214–1292
(Translation by R.B. Burke, 1928)

5

A fledgling nephrologist at McGill, 1961–1969

NEPHROLOGY WAS STILL AN EVOLVING FIELD of medicine when I took my post at McGill University in 1961, but little did I suspect that this evolution would launch a virtual revolution in another field: medical ethics.

It began in May 1962, when I attended the annual meeting of the American Society of Clinical Investigation in Atlantic City, New Jersey. As always, the atmosphere was exciting as well as competitive, and the quality of presentation was very high. But the highlight on this occasion was a presentation by Dr. Belding Scribner from Seattle. His research group had shown that the right time to use the artificial kidney (hemodialysis) for patients with acute kidney failure was *before* symptoms of renal failure (uremia) developed, not as a treatment for uremia *after* it had developed and was progressing. This was a novel claim and, at that time, constituted a breakthrough concept. It brought sharply to mind our hesitation to use hemodialysis before the identical-twin kidney transplant in 1958 (see Chapter 4); we believed that hemodialysis was a hazardous procedure, only to be used as a last resort. It is a curious testament to medicine's conservatism that dialysis was available for about ten years before this crucial aspect of its use was demonstrated.

The Scribner group showed that people with chronic renal failure could be kept alive and in good health, without appreciable urinary production, for a year or more with hemodialysis. This had never been done before. The abstract of their classic presentation reads as follows:

A new pumpless, low temperature hemodialysis system and a technique of long-term cannulation of blood vessels have been developed and perfected to the point where it is now possible to restore to good health selected young adults with chronic kidney disease who would otherwise die of terminal uremia. The first four patients were begun on a weekly hemodialysis during the winter of 1960. One of three patients, with a creatinine clearance of 1 mL per minute, continues to work full time. Two others, who have been anuric [absent urine secretion] for the last 18 months, lead comfortable sedentary lives. The fourth died of a myocardial infarction [heart attack] after a year of hemodialysis therapy. Hypertension, which became malignant in one patient, has been satisfactorily controlled solely by a low salt diet and ultrafiltration of extracellular fluid during dialysis. About a year ago, two of the four patients developed a slowly progressive peripheral neuropathy and all complained of uremic symptoms prior to each weekly dialysis. Switching from a long weekly dialysis of 16 hours to 12 hours of dialysis twice a week has resulted in elimination of predialysis symptoms and improvement in neuropathy.

In the last eight months, four additional patients have been added to the program. Each was carefully selected as being an emotionally stable, mature, cooperative adult under the age of 40 who was free of serious complications of hypertension. Each was suffering from terminal uremia (accumulation in the blood of constituents normally eliminated in the urine that produces a severe toxic condition) at the time treatment was begun. Hemodialysis once or twice weekly has restored each to good enough health to return to work; one patient married recently. All patients require weekly transfusions to prevent severe anemia. Accumulation of iron may present a potential threat. Exhaustion of cannula sites is another potential problem, but recent improvement in cannula design may have solved this problem.

It is concluded that selected young adults with terminal uremia can be restored to good health with periodic hemodialysis.[26]

Although scientific meetings are meant to be conducted in a matter-of-fact manner, with the presentation of evidence, drawing justifiable conclusions in a reasoned and logical manner of speaking, the effect of this dramatic result, so plainly put before us, was electrifying. Instead of the usual somewhat perfunctory applause, the entire audience—more than 2,000 physicians and researchers—rose as one and gave Scribner a warm, prolonged, standing ovation. It was simply a wonderful occasion! This presentation put long-term maintenance hemodialysis on the map as an effective treatment for chronic kidney failure. Interestingly, it also had other implications, particularly in the field of medical ethics.

The birth of contemporary bioethics

This initial demonstration that a person in chronic kidney failure could be kept well using an artificial kidney (maintenance hemodialysis) gave birth to the whole question of the allocation of scarce health resources. At the time, there were only two hemodialysis units in all of Canada and the cost of using them for this purpose was about $25,000 a year per patient. Could society afford this? No one knew for sure. How many would need it? A common estimate, then, was about 70 patients per million. This works out to a staggering figure—about 1,680 patients in Canada at that time. This scarcity of units in the face of overwhelming need boiled down to a question of who shall be saved when not all may be saved. The decision to accept some, but not all, for dialysis treatment became one of the major issues that stirred public and professional interest in medical ethics, and for the first time opened medical decision-making process to public scrutiny.

The Seattle group set up a committee, which included philosophers and theologians, to try to make the patient selection. This committee was later called the "God Squad" and their decision-making process was described in a famous *Life* magazine article.[27]

There had been resource allocation decisions before this time, of course. One only need think of the triage practiced in wartime when casualties were brought into a field dressing station. But under those dire conditions there was no time for ethical considerations; medical staff triaged according to status and urgency, allocating resources accordingly. In the case of dialysis, however, there was the time—and the need—to consider the question of allocation of resources. This captured the public interest and started a process that became increasingly complex as the advances of post-World War II medicine unfolded. Indeed, Dr. Al Jonsen, one of my gurus in medical ethics, dates the birth of modern medical ethics from this actual event,[28] and the poignant dilemmas that it raised during the decade before U.S. Congress legislation in 1972 amended the U.S. Social

Ethical Dilemma

The choice of who gets to go on dialysis rests mainly with the treating physician, not the hospital administrator, not the ministry of health (though their responsibility for additional resources is critical), and not the insurance company. Thus, a nephrologist might find him- or herself being both an advocate for their patients and the decision-maker for a dialysis program, which included other nephrologists' patients as well. This sets up an ethical conflict between "My principal duty is to advocate for my patient, under all circumstances" and "I and my colleagues have become gatekeepers for the use of this valuable but scarce resource, and we must choose." It is small wonder that there was a need for others to be involved.

Security Medicare plan, making it compulsory to provide hemodialysis to all people with chronic kidney failure.

The same dilemma was faced in Canada until 1968, when the publicly-funded universal health insurance plan for all medically necessary procedures came into effect. Clearly, this form of treatment was medically necessary for people with chronic kidney failure—it was the only means of prolonging their lives.

The Taguchi loop

It would be several years before long-term maintenance dialysis was available to everyone who needed it, even though units were being developed across the country, including at the Montreal General Hospital. In addition, it still was not fully accepted that people with chronic kidney failure could be effectively kept alive for years by dialysis, even though Scribner's group had shown that they could live for more than a year. This scepticism, combined with the cost of the treatment and the numbers who could potentially benefit, meant that research continued into alternative methods of getting rid of the nitrogenous end-products of the body's metabolism that the kidney normally excretes, including three main ones—urea, uric acid and creatinine.

Staff at the Royal Victoria Hospital (RVH), including myself, were among many exploring alternative approaches. We knew that transplantation would come one day soon, but we were also intrigued by the possibility that the lining of the gut could be used as a membrane for washing out the

Figure 5.1 Intestinal perfusion for kidney failure.

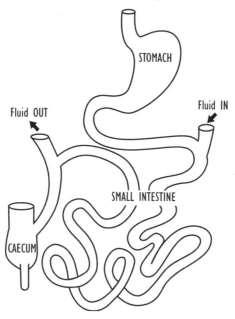

nitrogen end-products when the kidneys failed. It was known that urea, the main nitrogen end-product of the body, diffused easily through all cell membranes and all tissues; however it seemed doubtful that urea was the main toxic agent in kidney failure. The hope was that the other more toxic molecules could also be extracted by passing fluids through the intestine, and with a bit of time, these nitrogenous substances would diffuse from the body into the effluent fluid—that is, through "intestinal washout."

The main credit for this approach should go to Dr. Yoshinori Taguchi, then a resident on the urology service. His idea was to insert two tubes: one close to the top of the jejunum (the upper end of the small intestine), the other close to the end of the ileum (the last division of the small intestine), before it enters the large intestine or colon (Figure 5.1). The section of the small intestine between these two tubes could then be infused with a saline-like physiological solution, top to bottom, for four to eight hours each day. The idea was that the nitrogen end-products would diffuse out of the bowel wall into the perfusion fluid. The rest of the day, the whole bowel was left to perform its normal digestive functions.

In contrast to hemodialysis, this method was simple and inexpensive once the patient had been surgically prepared. Early results were encouraging: urea was readily removed and normal levels restored;

A fledgling nephrologist

acid/base and electrolyte disturbances were readily controlled. Patients tolerated the procedures and improved noticeably in the early weeks. We were encouraged and entered an abstract for the first meeting of the International Society Nephrology at Evian, France.

Unfortunately, in the months before the meeting, several patients who seemed to be doing very well died unexpectedly. We had noted that this procedure did not lower the quantity of two nitrogen end-products: uric acid and creatinine. In fact, these had steadily climbed in the patients' blood. At autopsy, we found an advanced arteriosclerosis (an obstruction of arteries) of medium- and small-sized arteries and crystals of urate (uric acid) in various tissues, notably in the heart. At these sites, urate deposits were associated with scarring. The patients had died of sudden heart failure.

We stopped the whole procedure after these findings. Six patients had undergone jejuno-ileal loop perfusion treatment for chronic kidney failure; unfortunately, none of them survived.[29]

Ethical Dilemma

Was this the right experiment to do? What could possibly justify it when Scribner had already shown that maintenance hemodialysis would provide complete substitution for kidney function for periods in excess of a year?

But, as explained above, once it had been shown that nitrogenous excretion could be achieved by simple diffusion exchange across a cellophane membrane (which is all that hemodialysis is), it was not unreasonable to look for a natural membrane (e.g., the lining of the small bowel) to use instead. This was a much less expensive option that could potentially be made available to everyone.

Unfortunately, the experiment was unsuccessful. The small bowel cannot be used as a simple diffusion membrane. Some people thought it was a worthless avenue to even pursue, and we were sensitive to their scornful criticism. I still feel much remorse for those who died in this project, regardless of how enthusiastic we were about it when we reported it in 1963 in the *Canadian Medical Association Journal*.[30]

Would our experiment have failed to pass the scrutiny of a research ethics board (REB)? That is a crucial question. I think the answer is that a REB, if they had existed then, might well have thrown objections in its way. To which one can make the following riposte: W.J. Kolff, who invented the artificial kidney in Holland in 1945, remarked that of the first 16 patients who used his machine, 15 died.[31] Much later, in the mid-1970s, he posed the question of whether he would have been allowed to go on with his research if there had been a REB. He replied: No, his research would have been stopped.

The flaw in our project—and this was equally a flaw in Kolff's research—is that it should first have been worked out in animals. If we had evidence that animals without kidneys could be maintained for some months by intestinal perfusion, then everything we did would have been ethically sound.

Another approach to the ethics of this project would be to consider it as an example of innovative treatment. This addresses the following question: When faced with imminent death or other catastrophe where there is no established medical therapy, is it ethical to try out a new idea—acting on a hunch, as it were—under the rubric of innovation, provided that

- the patient knows that it is only for his/her benefit (and therefore the doctors are not seeking generalizable knowledge—as would be the case if it was research), and
- the patient and other professionals—including nurses—give their consent?

Despite my obvious conflict of interest, I still think back on this approach to end-stage renal failure as a justifiable situation of innovative treatment for those six people in the early 1960s, although others may well disagree. The project was stopped the very day crystals of uric acid deposits were seen in the heart muscle during the autopsy of the first of these patients to die.

A windfall

Every now and then something truly remarkable happens that changes the course of one's career. The following case illustrates how dealing with another's vulnerability and disease may lead to incredible trust, gratitude and opportunity.

One Saturday morning, I was having a coffee in the urology department at the RVH with several surgeons and residents when the conversation drifted to discussion of unusual clinical situations. One of the senior urologists remarked: "You know, I felt sure it would be a calculus [kidney stone]—the colicky pain, the blood in the urine, some tenderness in the flank on deep palpation—but when I got up there with the retrograde ureteric grabber, all I could bring out was reddish pulp. No grittiness, no sign of stone. Quite odd!"

After several colleagues gave some desultory speculations, it occurred to me that he might have snagged a sloughed (dropped off) renal papillus in his ureteric grabber. (There are 15 to 20 renal papillae, small nipple-like internal projections in the kidney, where 200 to 300 collecting tubules for urine are gathered together in a bundle of ducts. Sometimes blood supply to these pyramids is affected and they die, then drop off.) A sloughed papillus could give the symptoms of a stone (see Figure 5.2).

As they left, I made a parting comment: "Why don't you ask him this question: 'How many bottles of pain pills would you say you get through in a month?' When he tells you, ask him: 'Do those contain the usual 15 to 20 per bottle, or do you always buy bottles of a hundred?' My hunch is that you may find his answers surprising!"

Early nephrologists saw disease of the renal papillus more often than urologists, and it was my experience that papillae may decay and fall away in the kidney disease that is associated with excessive intake of over-the-counter pain pills—especially when those pills contain phenacetin, although no one has ever adequately explained why this is so. After this cause of chronic renal failure was recognized in the late 1960s, pharmaceutical companies stopped selling phenacetin, but in 1968, when we reported 22 cases in Canada, the common analgesic preparation, Frosst 222, contained the offending compound.[32] The pills also contained codeine, which is of course why people liked taking them.

About an hour later, I was paged by the urologist. "Guess what!" he said. "The patient buys about four bottles a month, and always 100 tablets at a time!" We concluded that this was the source of the problem. The patient had phenacetin nephritis. The urologist was generous in telling the family that his nephrologist colleague had come up with the diagnosis, and they asked to meet me.

Some months later, this gentleman slipped into kidney failure and needed to be placed on dialysis. He became a patient under my care and I did what I could to make life bearable for him, including visiting him at home when things were not going well. I seemed to get on very well with the family and they certainly seemed to trust my judgement.

Figure 5.2 Cross section of a kidney.

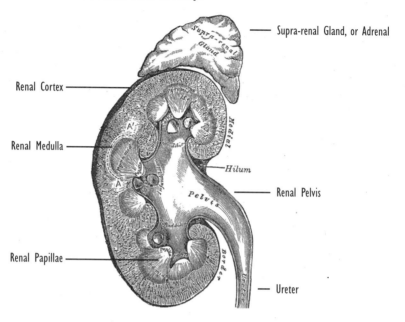

Supra-renal Gland, or Adrenal

Renal Cortex

Renal Medulla

Hilum

Renal Pelvis

Renal Papillae

Ureter

After he had been on dialysis for about a year, I got an emergency call when I was visiting the transplantation group at The Cleveland Clinic, to say that he had experienced a cardiac crisis and was dying. I immediately flew back to Montreal only to find that he had died. I felt bad, as I had promised to be there for this family with whom I had developed a special relationship. I felt I had let them down at the moment of greatest crisis.

Three months later, a young family member—now a family decision-maker—called and asked to see me. My first thought was that he wanted to tell me that the family grieved at my absence when his father died and I anticipated the need to apologize. But it was not that at all. The family wanted to know how they could use their wealth to promote research and treatment of kidney failure patients at the RVH—including building a kidney floor, if that was what was most needed. I was at a loss for words. I was truly bowled over.

After several meetings, the family agreed to build a small research laboratory to promote kidney transplant research, and finance two resident training and research positions for a five-year period, with a review of the nature of their continued support at the end of that time.

This made a tremendous difference to how the programs developed during the rest of my time at McGill. The strengthened infrastructure

Ethical Dilemma

Should wealth be a way to preferential care? Although I do not recall any anticipation of such immediate or massive financial help for our research program, I have since wondered why I gave this family so much more of my time than others. Did I show them special attention just because they were rich? Or was it because they were so very appreciative and friendly, and evoked a personal warm response on my part? Was it legitimate to promote the interests of one's patients and one's professional responsibility when an opportunity presents?

In Canada, their wealth made no difference whatsoever to my personal income—I am glad of that. At the time, I was funded on a full-time university salary, without the option of supplementation from private work.

Professional ethics would not permit a physician to have special patients in a publicly funded system such as Canada's. Yet one could partly justify showing special attention to the really wealthy in a society that embraces the capitalist ethos, if the ulterior motive was to ask them to strengthen a research program and increase the quality of care for all kidney failure patients through their individually-chosen generosity.

also favourably influenced our ability to obtain Medical Research Council (MRC) grants, as well as helping to secure my appointment to the status of a Career Investigator of the MRC, which later provided my salary for 15 years.

The ethics of disproportionate wealth and delivery of health care is a complex and recurring one. I experienced the dilemma in its sharpest poignancy when dealing with the question of kidney dialysis and transplantation in India.

In the 1960s, where was nephrology research in Canada?

I have tried to give a taste of what it was like to be one of this new breed of medical specialists—nephrologists—in Canada in the 1960s. For those whose kidneys had failed, and irreversibly so, there was now the hope of long-term maintenance dialysis and, perhaps, kidney transplantation. But where was the support for new research into expanding this field? It was nowhere, and it was clear that we needed specific research endeavours in nephrology.

Unfortunately, in medicine, it happens all too often that each step forward is prompted by human tragedy. This was true also for the founding of the Kidney Foundation of Canada, where the tragedy concerned the illness of Morty Tarder, a young architect in Montreal. In 1964, he developed renal failure as a result of a condition known as Goodpasture's Syndrome and came under my care. More recently, this condition would have been treated with Prednisone, Cyclophosphamide and extensive plasma exchanges (plasmapheresis) in order to remove harmful antibodies directed against vital cell structures in the kidneys and lung. However, in 1963 there was no plasmapheresis and little knowledge about the harmful auto-antibodies, except that there was a risk of lung hemorrhage, and that, therefore, the anti-coagulation involved with hemodialysis carried serious and special risks.

Some patients with this condition had spontaneous improvement, with resolution of the disease. Unfortunately, Morty Tarder was not to be one of these. When Morty died under my care at the Royal Victoria Hospital, his father, Harry Tarder, said in grief and despair, "Can't anything be done to prevent this sort of thing in this day and age? Surely someone can do something?"

I was deeply affected by his remark and a day or so later, I had an idea. I contacted my colleague at l'hôpital Hôtel Dieu de Montréal, Dr. Guy Lemieux, who was enthusiastic in his support. I asked to meet again with Mr. Tarder to discuss the possibility that he and his business associates, together with other people, might be able to act on his initial impulse of doing something to promote kidney research. This was the first step towards bringing to life the Kidney Foundation of Canada.

Progress was slow in the early years, but the support continued to grow. As I recall, only $3,000 was raised in the first year—but wonderful people supported the cause and the Kidney Foundation spread across Canada, with branches in every province. Suffice it to say that by the turn of the century, in addition to its many other activities, the KFOC research budget was $2 million, with many more millions in a support fund that could be drawn upon in lean years. The Foundation continues to go from strength to strength.*

---

* For more information, see the Kidney Foundation of Canada website at
  http://www.kidney.ca/index-eng.html.

As to the moral proprietary of prolonging life, we must keep it firmly in mind that...the benefactions of medicine express themselves in increasing life expectancy. This is virtually all that medication does, including the most ordinary pills and plasters, and it should be clearly understood that the difference between... everyday medications and...a heart-lung machine is a difference of degree only, not of principle. There is no philosophically definable dividing line between treatment that is rated dignified and morally acceptable and that which is declared to be an affront to the dignity of man.

How can we ever come to firm conclusions on any of this?... Opinions do take shape slowly though they are not rational in origin. I mean, they are not inferences from philosophic or theologic axioms or explicit guidance from Holy Writ: they are formed by the exercise of a sort of moral equivalent of the Common Law....

Moral consensus originates in the same way and I believe also that the moral consensus is just another heritage and, in my judgement, does not regard the support of life as the equivalent to prolongation of dying or in any way as an affront to human dignity or a diminishment of man.

Sir Peter Medawar (1915–1987)[33]
The Threat and the Glory: Reflections on Science and Scientists, 1991

6

Early experiences in kidney transplantation at McGill, 1963–1969

IN THE EARLY 1960s, while new techniques in nephrology and artificial kidney treatments (hemodialysis) were rapidly unfolding, transplantation was emerging as another option for patients with kidney disease, although there was much concern about the ethics of that enterprise.

Perhaps the largest concern in these early days was, and in most parts of the world still is, the question of how much money and other resources should be spent to extend the lives of a small number of people when there are so many other societal needs. In the early days, there were also ethical concerns over whether it was right to use organs from dead people, or whether it constituted a sort of sacrilege. Because the first transplant results were not very encouraging, some people wondered whether we were doing more harm than good and whether we should call a moratorium. (This was later done in two areas: xenotransplantation, following the publication of two reports in 1964,[34,35] and permanently implanted artificial hearts, after Barney Clark and the Jarvik-7 heart, in 1982.[36])

Despite these concerns in the early 1960s, the pressure of human suffering brooked no delay. No one knew if hemodialysis would prolong life over the long term, say, five to ten years, or whether transplantation would be the better long-term option, so it seemed ethically appropriate to pursue both options. Certainly, without dialysis as backup, it would not have been ethical to go into such an experimental field. There was also an urgent need to help people who did not have access to maintenance hemodialysis. At that time there were no chronic renal failure programs east of Montreal; we hoped renal transplantation would provide an option for those patients.

In 1963, we knew that most of the basic science questions around transplantation had not been answered—indeed, many still await solution in the third millennium—but scientists and physicians sensed that a new era in organ failure was dawning. Unlike earlier experiments, such as the intestinal loop perfusion (see Chapter 5), which was exclusively done on human subjects, basic and animal transplant experiments preceded human transplants. (Peter Medawar and colleagues had performed Nobel Prize-winning experiments on mice at Oxford in the 1950s.)

However, basic and animal research is not sufficient; knowledge also resides in clinical research. Basic immunologists (specialists in the immune system) were reluctant to proceed with kidney transplantation because they did not appreciate how different the kidney is from other organs. Nephrologists, on the other hand, were more optimistic. They knew that the kidneys, which normally receive about 25 per cent of the total output of blood from the heart, per beat or per minute, have an enormous blood flow but actually require relatively little blood to stay alive. Even acute renal failure patients who are without kidney function for several weeks can make a total recovery. During kidney shut-down, the very low residual blood flow (about 15 per cent) can keep the organ alive for three to five weeks, although it does not produce urine during that time. It is as if it is hibernating. Thus, nephrologists could predict that rejection in a kidney might be quite different than in a skin graft, because the kidney is not as vulnerable to sustained falls in blood flow. This understanding justified pursuing an alternative to dialysis for chronic kidney failure—namely, transplantation—and forging ahead at the clinical research level.

Sir Peter Medawar acknowledged this a decade and a half later in 1976 when, as president of the International Transplantation Society, I recall him saying something to the effect that, "If you clinicians had waited until the basic immunologists could say 'Well, we understand enough about the whole process for you to go ahead now with some clinical trials', you would still be waiting!"

Transplant pioneers

A cadaveric donation comes from a person who is brain dead, but whose vital organs are maintained artificially. The pioneering work in clinical cadaver kidney transplants came from Drs. Joseph Murray, John Merrill and colleagues at the Peter Bent Brigham Hospital in Boston. As a plastic surgeon, Murray had been drawn into the field of allogeneic skin grafts (grafts from other members of the same species), although it was clear that skin differed from solid organ grafts, which was the ultimate goal. Thus, when he was joined in 1960 by a young British research fellow and surgeon, Dr. Roy Calne, it was natural that experiments would be carried out with organs (kidneys) in dogs. Murray and Calne also had a new Burroughs Wellcome drug called azathioprine (Imuran) that was used in conjunction with prednisone, radiation and actinomycin C.[37] This animal work launched the era of transplantation. (Calne was knighted and became a professor of surgery at Cambridge University, while Murray was awarded a Nobel Prize in 1990 [shared with E. Donnell Thomas of Seattle, the pioneer in bone marrow transplants].)

This team showed that solid organs actually have some advantages over skin. Skin gets its blood supply mainly by diffusion from surrounding areas and sprouting of capillary blood vessels (angiogenesis). This delicate process makes skin much more sensitive to disruption by the inflammation of rejection than solid organs. With solid organs, the large blood vessels can be sewn together by the surgeon, immediately restoring blood flow to the grafted organ.

Their canine experiments were so successful that clinical protocols were undertaken within months.[38] When the Royal Victoria Hospital (RVH) decided to proceed with cadaveric kidney transplantation in 1963, these same protocols were used. It was just what we needed to get us off the mark.

I had the good fortune to be the physician who directed the medical aspects of this venture (in contrast to the surgical component). I worked with Dr. Lloyd McLean, chief of surgery, and Dr. Ken MacKinnon, chief of urology, with support from Dr. John Beck, who ran the metabolism service.

The early months were difficult. The fear of infection under the influence of immune suppressive drugs (especially azathioprine) was such that we felt the need to build three isolation rooms, each leading into a higher degree of protection against invasive bacteria: a scrub room, leading to a preparation room, leading to the room where the patient lay. It took about ten minutes to get into the inner sanctum. We arranged for specially purified air, and everything going into the suite was autoclaved (treated with steam under pressure) or boiled. The food was specially sterilized, even the patient's cigarettes were autoclaved and then dried out. Not surprisingly, patients expressed a strong aversion to such isolation. All this turned out to be unnecessarily cautious when it was later realized

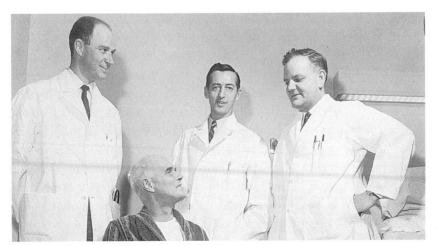

In 1963, the kidney transplant team at the RVH included (left to right) Dr. Lloyd MacLean, Dr. Ken MacKinnon and Dr. John Dossetor.

that there was no way the patients could be protected from the organisms that they carried in their bowel and on their own skin. As experience grew, the level of isolation became much more reasonable and less of a psychological strain on the patient and relatives, though the latter still had to gown, glove and mask when visiting.

In those early days, using kidneys from those who had just died—even with permission from relatives—was a repugnant concept to many people, including many of my medical colleagues in Montreal. I shared it myself, to some extent. But over time I came to look upon this act, that some saw as a *desecration* of the dead, as a *consecration* to life made possible by the altruism of the families who agreed to let others use the organs of their loved one so soon after they had been deprived of their presence. I saw this as an important ethical issue with which I am now very comfortable—recognizing that there are cultures (e.g., Japanese), and some religions, where this custom is still seen as a desecration.[*39]

In addition to this issue, cadaver transplantation also brought to the fore the question of when one could define the moment of death. The need to minimize the period of non-perfusion (when blood is not being pumped

---

* Although the 1997 Organ Transplant Law in Japan legalized organ procurement from brain-dead donors, the controversy surrounding this issue persists. Sixteen months elapsed between passage of the law and performance of the first legal heart, cornea, kidney, and liver transplant procedures using organs procured from a brain-dead donor.

Ethical Dilemma

The concept of death by cerebral criteria (brain death) is very important to transplantation. Before the transplant era, everyone accepted that death was associated with the cessation of breathing and heart beat. It did not matter which came first, both dysfunctions had to be present for a person to be dead. But, if organs were then going to be placed into other people, the quality of the transplanted organ became important. When someone's brain had been so severely injured that it was absolutely clear to the neurosurgeons and neurologists that there was no chance of survival, then it was thought death had occurred, even though the body was kept breathing with a ventilator, the heart was still beating, blood pressure was maintained, and kidneys, liver and bowel were still functioning.

This is especially so when the blood supply to the brain is cut off by a rapid rise in pressure within the skull (which occurs with brain swelling in response to injury). The most convincing evidence to support the fact that absence of brain blood flow for a period of time leads to brain autolysis (aseptic liquefaction) comes from a case where the body of a pregnant woman, following brain injury, was kept on life support for ten weeks, until delivery. At autopsy, the skull contents were liquefied, and the pathologist was able to see the upper part of the spinal cord when the vault of the skull was removed.[40]

After experiencing these situations several times, I too was convinced that such bodies were dead. They were no longer patients, they were lifeless bodies without brains but with beating hearts. The difficulty in believing that such bodies are dead is still experienced by those coming across the situation for the first time, especially since the diagnosis is not possible in comatose states due to drugs or hypothermia.

through the body's organs) made this a crucial issue. There was enormous pressure to clarify the term "brain death," which was becoming parlance.

With cadaveric transplantation becoming a clinical reality, new questions arose concerning who was suitable as a donor after death. This debate still continues. At McGill we made a number of mistakes, including:

- transferring breast cancer from a patient who had died of cerebral hemorrhage to the immunosuppressed kidney recipient;
- transferring toxoplasmosis (an infection that may seriously damage the central nervous system), which had been imperfectly diagnosed in the donor and that was not that person's primary cause of death; and
- implanting kidneys that had undergone a long period of low blood pressure before death, and subsequently did not function after implantation.

It was a learning curve for everyone, especially for a nephrologist—namely, myself—who was endeavouring to become a transplant physician. These were the mistakes of ignorance and we learned from them, but the question of moral guilt still lingers. Should we have been learning like this from experience with human subjects? How much could have been learned from animal models? Indeed, we had research programs in dogs to look at some of these questions, under the supervision of Lloyd MacLean and myself.

In retrospect I have to wonder whether the early transplantation efforts were premature. The first publication in Canada on the use of cadaveric kidneys was our paper in the *Canadian Medical Association Journal*[41] in 1964 on four patients: three died soon after transplantation, the fourth was still surviving after 18 months. Nowadays such results would be considered totally unacceptable and the program would be discontinued. At the time it was seen as part of a pioneering effort and results elsewhere were similarly poor. Most places were reporting one or two such transplants and then waiting to assess outcomes in the longer term. The largest early series of cadaveric transplants was at The Cleveland Clinic in Ohio; the second largest was ours in Montreal (though only for a short time).

Towards the end of 1963 the National Institutes of Health held a conference in Washington[42] where the results presented were so uniformly dismal that there was talk of a moratorium, especially on kidneys from live donor relatives, until complications were better understood.[*43] This view was shared widely until the bombshell from Colorado hit.

Bombshell from Colorado

This foreboding was blown away by the 1964 publication by Dr. Tom Starzl and his group at Denver, Colorado.[44] This very active group were

Ethical Dilemma

Can one restrict the decision-making capability of fully competent persons?

The series in their studies included 13 unrelated live donors, all of whom were males between the ages of 20 and 45. Normally, live donors are more likely to be mothers than fathers, and no one else was then reporting on unrelated living donors. Where, one asked oneself, would such a source of predominantly male, early middle-age altruists be found? It later turned out that they were prisoners in the Colorado State Penitentiary system. Starzl, in his autobiography *The Puzzle People*,[45] admits that he would now consider this source of donors to have been coerced, and the process unethical, but back then it seemed an acceptable trade-off: in exchange for a kidney, the prisoners were offered a commutation of their sentence.

This issue will resurface around the question of purchasing kidneys for transplantation. The ethical conflict is between recognizing and according to all competent individuals their *complete autonomy* in making decisions in their own interests, on one hand, and protecting individuals from being coerced into decisions, that do not, in the long run, serve either their own interests or those of the *common good*, on the other hand.

---

* Of 28 monozygotic twins who received transplant, 21 were living but seven had died. Of 91 who had received transplants from blood relatives, only five were alive after one year. Of 120 patients who received kidneys from unrelated live donors or from cadavers, only one survived for more than one year.

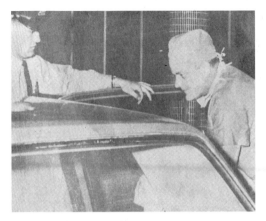
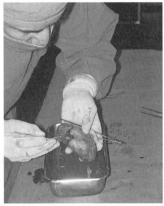

These two photos show aspects of a kidney transplant, using an organ from someone who had died in another hospital in Montreal in 1965. Here (left) the organ is carried from one hospital to the other with great care and speed in an ice-chilled solution. At the implanting hospital (right), the kidney is perfused with special solution and prepared for surgical implantation.

involved in transplanting kidneys from both cadaveric and live donors. Encouraged by their early results, they rapidly performed and reported 56 transplants—a larger experience than the rest of the world put together. Their results were good, but contained an ethical dilemma not much talked about at the time.

From the transplantation point of view, Starzl's results were a bombshell. He took kidney transplantation from clinical research to established procedure in a few short months. After his research was published, there was no more talk about moratoria, although there were still ethical concerns that cadaveric transplantation was not the best option for those in chronic renal failure; maintenance hemodialysis between 1963 and 1968 offered better patient survival.

We were able to refer patients who clearly would do well to the excellent hemodialysis program at the Montreal General Hospital. But we felt ethically justified in presenting the cadaveric and live related-donor transplant option to those for whom it was the best solution because of live donor availability, geography, or other factors. In the mid-1960s, there were two transplant units in Canada: ours and one at the University of Saskatchewan in Saskatoon (directed by Dr. Mark Baltzan). Patients were being referred to us for dialysis with a view to transplantation from as far away as the Atlantic Provinces and British Columbia.

Table 6.1 Values and principles used in resource allocations.

Rescue

those most in need should get priority

Utility

strive for the greatest good for the greatest number

illness prevention should be a priority

benefit should maximally outweigh burden (risk)

Equity

respond to need, not the ability to pay

resist pressure to serve the wealthy first

ensure that all have equal health entitlement

equalize opportunity when possible

Liberty

have freedom to exercise ability to pay

market forces make for cost-efficiency

Communitarianism

recognize community norms and standards

recognize relational interdependence

respect and promote social solidarity

Restitution

restore inherent rights/entitlements

compensate for past injustice

Worthiness (blameworthiness)

recognize social worthiness

reward good lifestyle

reward achievement

Lottery principle

first come, first served

recognize time spent on the waiting list

draw out of a hat (random choice)

Flawed values

the squeaky wheel gets the grease

bribery, the lobby, the media

nepotism, favouritism

blatant use of power

inappropriate fiduciary relations

Rationing

The R-word is dreaded in health care, yet it is present in many ways at various levels. Earlier, we encountered the principle in the "God Squad," which selected people for dialysis in Seattle in 1962. It was similarly an issue in the distribution of cadaveric organs for transplantation.

The need for rationing in transplantation, given the limited supply of cadaveric organs, becomes more critical each year. At this juncture, I will merely list the principles used to decide who should receive an organ (Table 6.1). Clearly, it is not an easy matter. Whose values are used? Who owns the organs after removal? Who has the authority to make these rationing decisions? Who should have this authority? Are physicians the most suitable people for this? Can the distribution be made fairer? These are weighty questions.

CASE STUDY: THE BOY UNDER THE BED

For J.K. [initials have been changed], transplantation was the preferred treatment. Indeed, it became the only option. This nine-year-old, who had been referred from Plattsburg, New York, had congenital abnormalities in his ureters and bladder that eventually led to chronic kidney failure. In his case, access sites into his body for hemodialysis had been used up quickly. There were no more sites in his arms for implantation of teflon-silastic shunts (the method of shunting blood from artery to vein, making a loop that could be opened for connection to the dialysis machine twice or three times a week); one leg's posterior tibial artery had also been used. Dialysis was being carried out through the remaining leg site, which was intermittently infected. His calf was tender with bluish discolouration, and he stood with this foot extended, walking on the balls of his toes. He was in pain, malnourished and miserable. His condition seemed to be leading inevitably to transplantation so he was placed on the list. Unfortunately, there was no suitable donor.

He hated and dreaded dialysis, and was so terrified of us that, anticipating our arrival on ward rounds, he would get out of his bed and disappear under it, crouching up against the wall. J.K. came to spend Christmas day with us that year and my family remembers him as a boy who was unhappy, weak, thin, irritable, and walking with a limp.

We were concerned about treating him against his will. He certainly did not "assent" to treatment. For this reason, several nurses challenged us, saying he should not be forced against his will, even though he would die without dialysis. We took these observations very seriously. Our response was not to stop dialysis and let uremia take over, but to place him on highest priority for

a transplant. This came up in a few months and was successful. He rapidly regained weight, vigour and his sense of well-being. Life became fun for him again, which was great to see.

I heard from his mother about ten years later. She described him as a surfing bum, somewhere on the beaches of California, in good health. But that little boy, crouching under his bed against the wall, haunts me still.

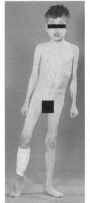
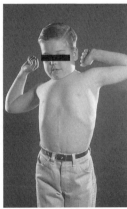

The boy under the bed: what a difference six months of kidney function can make.

BEYOND THE HIPPOCRATIC OATH

Ethical Dilemma

Should we go on treating a child who cannot consent, and does not assent? I do not believe we can ever give up on a young person if there is even a remote chance of restoring health and well-being, provided parents agree. But the poignancy of the situation is not difficult to imagine and there is room for much debate about these issues. If the person is an adult and fully competent, then we are bound, I contend, by the wishes of that person and no one else. To do otherwise would constitute assault or battery.

An unexpected finding from repeated exposures to another's blood

An unusual observation came out of the early kidney transplants. At that time, most people who underwent transplantation had been treated for months or even years on hemodialysis, during which they had many blood transfusions. This was particularly so in the early years because the first dialysis systems had to be primed with two sacs of blood (from different donors with compatible blood types). Because a patient underwent dialysis twice weekly, within six months they would receive blood from about 100 donors. We expected that these people would progressively become more sensitized (adversely react) to various white blood cell (leukocyte) factors they had received. Surprisingly, most did not.

Most people are familiar with the ABO blood group system.[*] If you receive the wrong type of blood, you will have an adverse reaction. There is also another set of factors—attached to the human leukocyte-A (HLA) system—which can cause an adverse reaction and, in the case of transplantation, rejection of the donor organ. There are about 60 different HLA factors, and each person carries eight of them. Although they are evident throughout the body's tissues, they are most readily assessed on leukocytes (white blood cells).

Our kidney patients on dialysis would receive myriad HLA factors from the blood that was used during the course of their treatment. Some, if not all, of those factors would be different from the eight that they had

---

[*] A type A recipient can receive a donation from type A or type O donors; a type B recipient can receive a donation from type B or type O donors; a type AB recipient can receive a donation from anyone—type A, B, AB or O donors; a type O recipient can only receive a donation from a type O donor.

on their own leukocytes. Normally, one would expect that they would become sensitized to the foreign factors. In other words, they would develop an immunological response (circulating antibodies or specific "killer" lymphocytes) to foreign material and reject any tissue (e.g., blood, organs) that contained them.

Why did our dialysis patients who had been exposed to many foreign HLA factors not have massive tissue sensitization and reject all kidneys right away? We reported on this[46] and it was subsequently widely cited, although we never discovered the reason for this. The reason—never proved—is that massive exposure to another person's tissue factors, entirely by the intravenous route, does not elicit immunity to the same extent that is associated with exposure by injection under the skin or in a muscle. Thus, the route by which these foreign HLA factors reach the recipient's immune system may be crucial. Even more curious was our observation that the more blood a person was exposed to during dialysis, the less likely he or she was to reject a subsequent cadaveric kidney transplant.

It seems that blood transfusions given to renal failure patients on dialysis who are awaiting transplant *favour* subsequent graft survival. We speculated that the overload of foreign HLA factors by the intravenous route induced partial immunological tolerance—a state of suppressed ability to respond immunologically to foreign factors (antigens). In other words, when a body is flooded with blood, it becomes overwhelmed by the variety of foreign HLA factors on the foreign white blood cells and turns off its response. It was a fine theory, but we did not then have to tools to test it.

However, there were clinical applications. We began requiring all transplantation patients to undergo at least six months of dialysis, thereby increasing their chance of accepting the donor organ. This finding also led to a number of research avenues, such as preplanned blood transfusions from a live related donor to the recipient during the weeks or months before kidney transplantation (thus exposing them to the HLA factors that would eventually be present in the donated kidney), and administering primitive donor bone marrow cells to recipients before transplantation.

Our findings also provided justification for the following unique professional experience.

CASE STUDY: A CHALLENGE FROM NEWFOUNDLAND

A doctor in Newfoundland phoned me about a woman in her mid-30s in renal failure whom he wished to refer to Montreal. She lived in a small fishing village on the south coast of the Rock, with her husband and five children. I responded from a simple *utilitarian** viewpoint, saying that follow-up after transplant would be impossible (at that time in winter, her village was only readily accessible by sea, and then only when the weather permitted). I said that we really could not manage her and that he should prepare them for the bleak outcome. But he was a *deontologist*.§ He placed her on the next plane with a polite little note asking us to "Please see and advise." How I now admire that man!

So we had this young woman on our ward and did not know what to do with her. We collectively decided that she could not be offered that very scarce resource, a cadaver kidney, because we knew we could not carry out our follow-up routines without which we deemed we would be acting irresponsibly and depriving someone else who could be appropriately followed-up of an opportunity. Reluctantly, we decided to give her peritoneal dialysis then transfer her back home, knowing she would die in a few weeks. But that fate was no different to the vast majority of renal failure patients at that time throughout Canada.

Then a remarkable fact was brought to my attention by one of the trainee residents on the service. There was another woman, in her 40s, in the same general medical ward who was dying of liver failure. By chance, she had the same blood type as the woman from Newfoundland. Our liver specialist, Dr. Alex Aranof,† had nothing further to offer the patient suffering from liver failure.

We conjectured that the following course of action, though very unusual, was justifiable—especially in light of our experience with blood transfusions. We figured that if the women were exposed to one another's HLA factors, they would develop immunological tolerance to those factors and thus, if transplantation later became necessary, the chance of success would be greatly

* Utilitarianism: making decisions that bring the greatest happiness or good to the largest number of people.

§ Deontology: the pursuit of good for each individual because each person is a moral equal and has value that is beyond price.

† It was Alec Aranof whom I had consulted about McGill and the RVH when Prof. Christie gave me 24 hours to make up my mind about coming to Canada in 1955! Alec was studying at the Post-Graduate Medical School in Hammersmith, London, and I had first met him there.

Figure 6.1 Diagram of cross-circulation between two persons, one with liver failure, the other with renal failure.

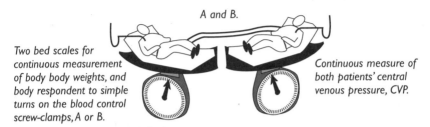

A and B.

Two bed scales for continuous measurement of body body weights, and body respondent to simple turns on the blood control screw-clamps, A or B.

Continuous measure of both patients' central venous pressure, CVP.

enhanced. (The practice of tissue typing—matching for the HLA factors—was not yet in common practice at the clinical level.)

With the consent of the patient with kidney failure and the family of the patient with liver failure, each of these patients agreed to have their two circulations linked artificially on an intermittent basis, so that each would have the use of the vital organ they lacked from the other (Figure 6.1). In other words, they could live in symbiosis by means of periodic cross-circulation for as long as was possible. It was possible that this could last for months, or even years. However, in the event of one dying, the vital organ that the other lacked would be available for post-mortem transplantation to the survivor. There was an elaborate consent document and full discussion of possibilities, even though most of the risks were unknown.

This was the first experience of cross-circulation between patients with different deficient organs, and it was extraordinary. The two circulations were intermingled using artery-to-vein silastic tube connections. The radial artery (just below the bend in the elbow) of one patient was connected to the brachial vein (upper arm) of the other. The volume of both circulations were kept constant using two balance beds and regulating the balance of body weights with a simple screw clamp on one of the silastic connecting lines.

In the course of a few hours, both subjects became fully conscious. The uremic patient did become transiently jaundiced because her liver excreted the accumulated bile pigment of the other, and the jaundiced patient had a brisk diuresis as her kidneys excreted the retained urea of the uremic patient. Both had identical hemoglobins, white blood counts, and electrolyte concentrations in the blood.

The experience was repeated several times over the next two or three weeks, each time cross-circulating for about 12 hours. Between episodes of cross-circulation, the silastic loop was reconstituted, artery to its own vein, in each person, so that they lived separate lives again.

We had no idea how to proceed with a longer term arrangement, but these negotiations were cut short when the cirrhotic patient suddenly died from a severe bowel hemorrhage. Fortunately, they were not in symbiotic cross circulation when this tragedy occurred. Unfortunately, it was Labour Day weekend and our surgeon was on holiday in Algonquin Park, Ontario. We used the RCMP to track him and get him back to Montreal, where he transplanted the kidney to the woman from Newfoundland.

The kidney did not function for two weeks, but it gradually "opened up" and began working normally. During that two-week period, I felt very awkward about the innovative research experience that we had all been through. Had we been carried away by the extraordinary coincidence of the blood group similarities of these two patients? To what extent were we motivated by the sheer excitement of putting our own observations of the possibility of creating immunologic tolerance by exposure to the foreignness of a donated organ to such a challenging test? My colleagues questioned me about what they had heard had been going on. They felt that we had gone too far and that the innovative treatment, though fascinating, had exceeded the bounds of the ethical. I was beginning to wonder if they were right.

But then the function of the transplanted kidney came back and the situation seemed more and more justified as each day dawned. I had a sense of great personal relief and delight in the improved health of our patient. After a month, the transplanted kidney was working well, and the woman was feeling well and planning her return to Newfoundland. She never experienced any significant rejection episodes on standard (in 1966) immunosuppression drug therapy. We speculated about the ultimate outcome. If multiple blood transfusions helped prevent rejection, then actual cross-circulation with an eventual donor should be even better.

She was subsequently seen at six month intervals. A year later, she became pregnant* and named her newborn daughter Victoria, after the hospital. The patient lived for another nine years and then died from a complication of imperfectly controlled hypertension.

---

* This was not the first of our transplanted patients to become pregnant. We believe another of our patients had the first such pregnancy in the world in 1964.

Ethical Dilemma

If one thinks through all the phases of this very unusual story, one cannot help but be struck by the succession of ethical dilemmas. They are truly daunting. Each ethical dilemma is highly defined by its actual context and influenced decision-making at the subsequent dilemma. We were moving into uncharted territory, and the trusting relationships between all involved were crucial. The issues include:

- medical and professional hubris;
- issues of saving a life at any cost;
- obtaining informed consent when no one knows the likely outcome;
- the absence of any outside ethical review;
- the complex nature of professional trust for those who are acting both as physician and investigator;
- the nature of personal respect; and
- the extraordinary fabric of the physician-patient relationship.

It is interesting to note that a similar case arose some years later and the proposal for cross-circulation was turned down by the newly instituted ethics committee.

These two cases were not the norm as we prepared people with chronic renal failure for cadaveric kidney transplantation. Typically, a man or woman in renal failure would live some distance from Montreal, be between the ages of 30 and 45, and have elected the RVH program of "dialysis with a view to transplant" over "maintenance dialysis in Montreal, without the option for transplant" at the other English-speaking hospital.

There were many such patients. We performed approximately 200 transplants between 1963 and 1970. The success rate for transplantation was gradually improving and many patients who lived in Montreal, for whom some would stoutly claim that maintenance long-term dialysis was the right treatment, nevertheless chose the transplant route.

Ethical Dilemma

This brings up the question of how to be fair when offering a choice between or among therapies. It has since bothered me that we did not use an impartial third party to offer the choice to our patients. How sure can I be that we did not unintentionally influence their decision in favour of the transplant route? There is no way to be sure.

A poll was taken among the Montreal General hemodialysis patients, asking them if they wanted to go the transplant route and almost all said they wanted to continue in their own program. But, were they, as a group, uninfluenced by the fact that they were in a non-transplant program, and did not want to disappoint those in charge of it? No one can say.

As in so many ethical dilemmas, there is no clear answer. For the individual patient, everything should hinge on the care with the patient is exposed to all the facts, hopefully by disinterested but fully informed third parties.

This ethical concern bedevils dialysis units into this millennium. The phenomenon is called "trapped in dialysis." Several studies have shown that American dialysis units where the profit motive is operating have a lower percentage of patients on transplant waiting lists than units in public institutions.[47] Is it because the patients are treated so well and given such individual attention that they are content to remain on dialysis and not be assessed for transplantation, or is it because there is a financial interest in not referring them to another form of treatment? Or is it both possibilities?

Nephrologist-cum-immunologist

Another difficulty that beset the early days of clinical transplantation was the absence of experts in clinical transplant immunology. As nephrologists like myself stumbled about in this new field, it was evident that knowing about renal physiology, electrolyte and acid/base problems, and how to give new immunosuppressive drugs was not enough. We had originally thought that the clinical immunologists would be able to help us out, but after reviewing a number of our problems, their frank response was that these were not the sort of allergic and auto-immune processes on which their immunology was based. They said we would have to develop our own immunologic awareness in this area. They were right, but it was a bit of a letdown just the same.

In addition to delayed-type immune reactions (those that took several days to evolve, mediated by specifically trained "killer cells"), we also had to cope with acute immune reactions (those taking minutes or hours to evolve, mediated by circulating "antibody" molecules). One of these acute reactions was seen when patients developed antibodies against HLA factors. As already mentioned, to a great extent we had been able to disregard the risks of possible tissue-borne sensitization to HLA factors during hemodialysis. In fact, we believed that we had even turned that possible risk into an advantage. But this was a fool's paradise. Before long, we realized that sensitization to HLA factors *did* occur in some of our patients. We stumbled across this sensitization process by chance. It turned out that it was also just at the right moment.

A serum test of immunosuppression
Dr. Jung (Jack) Oh, a research fellow from Korea, was trying to work out a method for measuring the immunosuppressive effects of azathioprine (at that time, the main anti-rejection drug) using blood serum (the clear yellowish fluid that remains after blood cells, fibrinogen and fibrin are removed from the blood) from transplant patients who were taking the drug. He began testing these serum samples against white blood cells (lymphocytes) in the hope that this would provide a means of standardizing the administration of the drug. He used serum from patients on hemodialysis as controls because they had never been exposed to azathioprine. As happens so often in research, things did not turn out as planned. First, some of the dialysis patients had serum that killed lymphocytes; second, in some, azathioprine had no effect on lymphocytes. But why?

Oh quickly worked out that it was the presence of antibodies in serum that was toxic to lymphocytes. It had nothing to do with azathioprine. These antibodies were found in three groups of people: healthy married women who had had a number of pregnancies; patients who had had a previously rejected transplanted kidney; and patients in whom blood from transfusions had leaked into tissues (i.e., had not been confined to the blood system), such as can occur after severe accidents.

Many women who have had several children are sensitized to their husband's HLA factors. The husband's HLA factors are introduced into the women's bodies through the fetus—which inherits half its blood factors from the mother, half from the father—via the placenta. Over the course of several pregnancies, these women develop a immunological intolerance to their husbands' HLA factors. The uterus provides an immunologic barrier to the mothers' antibodies so they have no effect on the fetus—even though it is the fetus that stimulates their formation. It is a fact that women with such antibodies (a majority of women who have had more than four children) will *acutely* reject their husband's skin if it is placed on their skin. These women are "loaded"—or pre-sensitized—to the lymphocyte factors that they do not share with their husbands.[*]

A dramatic example of what this can lead to occurred at the Montreal General Hospital in the early 1960s, when a husband donated a kidney to his wife who was in renal failure and on dialysis. To everyone's shock and dismay, the kidney turned black on the operating table. It was obviously not going to survive and had to be removed within minutes of implantation. The woman's antibodies had instantly started to attack the lining cells of her new kidney's blood vessels and destroyed it.

This phenomenon, which Oh had stumbled upon in his research, turned out to have great clinical significance in transplantation (although it could not be used to measure the effect of circulating azathioprine, as he had originally hoped). Awareness of these pre-formed antibodies to HLA factors quickly led to the understanding that one must test the serum of any potential transplant recipient against the cells of a potential donor (white blood cells are the most convenient cell to use). The test became the pre-transplant lymphocytotoxicity "cross-match" test, and has been used ever since. Our group discovered this cross-match test at more or less the same time as several other centres, independent of them all, but the scientific priority rightly goes to the Danish hematologist, Dr. F. Kissmeyer-Niehlsen.[48]

As it happens, the test came just in time; it saved us from taking a kidney from a leading Canadian politician to give to his son, who was on

---

[*] Lymphocytes are round white cells in the blood, lymph nodes and spleen that are the cellular mediators of immunity and make up 20 to 30 per cent of the white blood cells of normal human blood.

dialysis in Montreal. It would have been disastrous if we had gone ahead, but Oh's research revealed that the son's serum reacted with many people's white cells, including those from his father. We did not fully realize what this meant when it was first observed, so we decided not to proceed until we could figure it out. That took another year or so, by which time the young man had received a kidney from a cadaver donor and was doing well.

Learning transplant immunology was very difficult, but many surgeons became very proficient in the field as time went by, becoming what was later termed immunosurgeons. Such notables included Drs. Tom Starzl, Roy Calne, David Hume and Peter Morris.

Anti-lymphocyte serum: *Le Coup de Cheval*

In 1966 or so, a new method of controlling rejection arrived on the scene. Rather than chemical drugs, we tried to develop biologic factors—recently discovered for animal transplants—using antibodies against human lymphocytes to inhibit the body's immune reaction to a kidney bearing foreign HLA factors. Lymphocyte cells, which originate from stem cells and then differentiate, are cellular mediators of immunity, making up 20 to 30 per cent of the white blood cells. The hypothesis, then shown only in animal experiments, was that anti-serum containing antibodies to the recipient's lymphocytes would prolong graft survival. In other words, kill the killer lymphocytes before they kill the graft.

Anti-lymphocyte serum was made by injecting human lymphocytes into the tissues of animals (horses or rabbits). These animals then develop antibodies in their serum to the foreign lymphocytes, which inhibits rejection activity. When this serum is injected intra-muscularly into patients it was painful—hence the term *Coup de Cheval*.

There were two immediate problems: first, there was no commercial source of anti-lymphocyte serum to human tissue factors; and second, there was no standard by which to judge its potency. Despite this, and driven by poor clinical results in transplantation, a number of transplant centres decided to make the anti-lymphocyte serum for themselves. Montreal was no exception.

The reader's credulity will now be strained by the crudeness of our approach. Let me point out that transplantation research was still in its early days and there were still no research ethics review boards (they did not appear until about 1967). Clearly, you will be thinking that I am about to defend my ethics yet again, and I do not feel comfortable about it. You are right, but life *is* a bit rugged on the frontier.

The method used in Montreal was as follows: under my arrangements, Dr. Douglas Ackman, then a resident in urology working on the transplant service, collected human thymus material from the operating room (it was necessary to remove part of the thymus gland—the birthplace and training school for T-lymphocytes—when surgeons were operating behind the sternum on children to repair congenital defects in the heart). Thymus cells were made into a preparation that was injected into horses.

The horses belonged to one of the physicians at the RVH who had a farm, but stabled two of them at the McGill Agricultural College. The horses were resentful, no doubt, of the painful injection of human thymocytes (made more so by being mixed with Freund's adjuvant, a glue-like material calculated to increase antibody production). Nevertheless they dutifully made antibodies to human lymphocytes, which we then harvested, purified into gamma-globulin in our own research laboratory, and injected into patients as anti-lymphocyte globulin (ALG).

In retrospect, I tremble at our daring and foolhardiness. It was yet another example where I became involved enthusiastically in a clinical research program without really thinking out the possible ethical and legal traps, and without anyone from the outside questioning my actions. They might well have concluded that there is no justification for gambling in clinical research when people's well-being is involved, even if they have a fatal disease of an essential organ. To this, I might have replied, "Is it still gambling when their deaths are inevitable unless something new comes on the scene to help them?" But that still does not resolve the issue.

All clinical research has to be justified, but the rules for internal assessment were not well thought out or defined at this time. Nor did we have procedures in place for third-party screening of research protocols. I am also loath to admit that we did not even obtain permission from the parents of the children to use their thymus tissue for research because it was "discarded tissue." Once again, sensitivity to what would now be considered ethically essential was still far away.

The Medical Research Council steps up to the plate

Fate was to prevent us from getting into too much trouble over this, and from finding out if our homemade ALG really worked. Certainly, though painful when injected, ALG did not cause harm, and may have been

Ethical Dilemma

How does one tell when it is okay to go ahead with a new idea? I have spent a lot of time deliberating on this. One test for ethical propriety is: "If what you are about to do is of such a nature that you would be quite happy to have it reported on the front page of the local newspaper, then go ahead. If it is *not*, think again and act differently." This is acceptable because it holds one to a high community standard and that is what ethics is about—the word derives from the Greek word for customs or prevailing norms (*Ethos*).

Obviously, when dealing with historic events, this axiom must be modified: "If what you *did* was of such a nature that you would have been quite happy to have had it reported in the local press, then you were right to go ahead." Using the newspaper publication barometer, I would have deemed the above-mentioned research acceptable.

However, nowadays there is a third form of this axiom, and this is where the problem becomes troubling. Nowadays we would ask: "If what you did then *was* of such a nature that, *in the light of today's ethical perspectives*, you would still be quite happy to have had it reported on in the local newspaper, then it was right to go ahead. If it *would not be*, then you probably should have anticipated what could have happened and acted differently!"

In relation to our amateurish manufacture of anti-lymphocyte serum, my answer to this third question would be no. But hold judgement until you read the problems that the Medical Research Council (MRC) and Connaught Laboratories got into when they tried to do the same thing as we had done, so crudely, down on our farm.

Most ethicists would hold that the second form of the question is more crucial, but the third form is much more exacting and cannot be ignored. I suppose another yardstick—on the question of whether decisions made in the past were ethically appropriate—is to ask the question: "If exactly the same set of circumstances recurred, would you make the same decisions." The answer to both situations above—cross-circulation, and making one's own anti-lymphocyte globulin (ALG)—would be yes, but that is said with the knowledge that the exact circumstances cannot ever be repeated because of the progress of events on so many fronts. That question becomes moot.

helpful. But we never used enough of it to determine if it was effective against rejection, and no publications resulted from our research. It soon became clear that this was not the right way to go about developing an anti-lymphocyte serum. I was able to persuade people at the MRC in Ottawa that they should make an ALG that could be used in Canada and then run a multi-centre trial. The first step in this regard was a conference at McGill in 1967 on ALG. Experts from all over the world were invited to this MRC-sponsored two-day conference to discuss the new agent.

After this conference, the MRC financed production of anti-thymocyte globulin (ATG), contracting its production to Connaught Laboratories in Toronto. The MRC also arranged a conference of transplant physicians in Ottawa to plan a multi-centre trial of ATG in Canada. Unfortunately, the first 100 litres (and the first $100,000) had to be discarded because it contained an antibody to a protein in the base of many cells—the basement membrane—which would have destroyed kidney grafts directly. Beads of perspiration break out on my brow as I contemplate what would have been my fate if the McGill horse serum had been contaminated by the same antibody. There, but for the grace of God, a promising career—my own—would have gone down the tube. The second batch of MRC-sponsored ATG was okay, and was used in the multi-centre trial with success across Canada, although there were many delays and the paper on its use was not published until 1976.[49]

Makers of biologicals were very wary of getting into production of ALG or ATG serum. There was the question of standardization: one needed a large clinical trial to establish the correct dose, and that dose would only be correct for that particular batch of serum. Then there was the question of safety. Who knows what else might be included, either as an unwanted antibody (as in the first MRC batch) or viruses (hepatitis B had become detectable in that era, but non-A, non-B hepatitis—now known as hepatitis C—was not; other viruses were suspected, though not detectable).

A cautionary tale

The manufacturing vacuum for ALG led to a very strange situation in the University of Minnesota in Minneapolis. This was only partially settled by the university on November 17, 1997—20 years later—when it paid the U.S. federal government $32 million.

In 1970, researchers in Minneapolis, led by Dr. John Najarian, a world-famous transplant surgeon, and Dr. Fritz Bach started to manufacturer rabbit ALG with an investigational new drug order from the U.S. Food and Drug Administration (FDA). The enterprise prospered. The material was safe and effective and was used in more than 70 transplant centres, including a number in Canada. Manufacturing this quantity of ALG required the formation of a large private company. The problem was that the company never obtained FDA approval for distributing and selling the material after it had been shown to be safe and effective. More than $80 million in ALG sales were made without FDA approval. Further, the manufacturers had used tens of millions of dollars of National Institutes of Health (federal government) research funds to develop the product.[50]

In 1993, Najarian and a colleague, Dr. Richard Condie, were heavily compromised by all this. Condie, who ran the ALG program from 1971 to 1992, pleaded guilty to fraud, embezzlement and tax evasion, and then consented to testify against Najarian. In February 1996, Najarian, then president of the (international) Transplantation Society, was acquitted of all charges.[51] Happily he remains one of the "greats" in transplantation surgery.

It is hard to draw conclusions from this extraordinary matter, except that it shows the delicate path that the university researcher treads when he (or she) combines scientific progress with the for-profit ethos. Clearly it got out of control, but apportioning fair blame would be a research project in itself.

A change of direction
In 1968, as we were developing an interest in using ALG in transplantation, my professional life was developing in all sorts of directions, although transplantation immunology was coming to dominate. I was made a Career Investigator of the MRC, which I considered a great honour. Not only did this award pay my salary for five years, it also gave me "protected time" for research—over 50 per cent of my working hours— though I was permitted to continue seeing patients within my area of special competence. This award also had the unusual advantage of being transferable to other Canadian universities, in the event that I might decide to move. In due course, that is what happened.

My MRC research grant—an award separate from the Career Investigatorship—came up for review and, as was the custom, two people came to the RVH to discuss my research and plans for the future. This was a great privilege. In particular I valued the expertise of Dr. Frank Dixon, an experimental nephro-immunologist from the La Jolla Institute in California and a world figure in immunology. He said to me, in effect, that I either had to fish or cut bait. He said I could not go on indefinitely bearing the clinical load of a growing clinical transplant program—even though I had some wonderful physician support—and also expect to make significant progress in this new field of research. Which is it going to be, he asked, research or clinical practice?

It so happens that, around that time, my friend and nephrology colleague, Dr. Lionel McLeod, left the University of Alberta, where he was in charge of the Renal Division, to become physician-in-chief and head of the Department of Medicine at the University of Calgary. So the University of Alberta was looking for a replacement, and both Dr. Don Wilson, the chief of medicine, and Dr. Walter MacKenzie, the dean, wrote and visited me in Montreal, wondering if I would move to Edmonton.

I did not want leave McGill, even though the separatist movement in Quebec was beginning to make Anglophones a bit uneasy. But were those in charge at McGill prepared to make a special effort to support my desire to restructure my career along the lines that Frank Dixon had suggested? I wrote "Plans for the future" documents, consulted with Malcolm Brown in Ottawa, pressured the heads of surgery and urology—both of whom knew I had an offer from Edmonton in my briefcase—but all to no avail.

I think there was genuine surprise—though there should not have been—when I announced on January 1, 1969, that I would move to Edmonton on July 1. I had, of course, been discussing the possibility of the move with Margaret and the family, and Margaret had come out with me to Edmonton at Wilson's express invitation to look things over. I had also had a chance to meet Alberta's health minister, who made an unusual commitment. He promised to give me a fully-equipped transplantation laboratory (valued at $270,000) if the plan for a MRC (Ottawa) Transplant Unit did not come through. Thus, I was offered more that I had asked for at the Edmonton end, and nothing new at the McGill end. I guess that made the move inevitable.

As I reflect on the eight years I spent back at McGill, I realize how truly valuable, and career-forming, they were. In many respects, I was in the right place at the right time, at the cusp of a revolution in nephrology. But it was more than that: RVH and McGill supported and encouraged our efforts, celebrated our successes. And so it was not without some regret that I left Montreal in 1969.

SAY not the struggle naught availeth,
The labour and the wounds are vain,
The enemy faints not, nor faileth,
And as things have been they remain...
For not by eastern windows only,
When daylight comes, comes in the light;
In front the sun climbs slow, how slowly!
But westward, look, the land is bright!

—Arthur Hugh Clough (1819–1861)
Quoted by Winston Churchill, when
the U.S. entered World War II, following
the bombing of Pearl Harbor on Dec. 6, 1941

7

Research at the University of Alberta, 1971–1982

THE PROSPECT OF NEW CHALLENGES in a new city in Canada's remote West filled me with a spirit of adventure and excitement. My enthusiasm increased as I drove across the country in a sporty new Fiat 850 convertible. Of course, at a cost of $2,000, it was only a pseudo-sports car, but it was thrilling nonetheless. My high spirits persisted for the first few days after my arrival in Edmonton. I went into the office on July 2 and took it as being quite natural, quite *de rigeur*, that my new secretary, Kathy Dawe, would be decked out in a purple taffeta miniskirt with open-lattice black stockings and a feather in her heaped-up hair. It was, of course, Klondike Days—Edmontonians' celebration of their gold rush heritage—but as far as I knew, this was the way of the West. I mused to myself, "We're a long way from the Royal Victoria Hospital!"

I had left my wife and four children—Frances then 12, nine-year-old twins John and Clare, and Moira, age six—in Montreal because we had not sold the house (and would not do so for two years because of the political unrest at the time). The plan was that I would settle in for six months, then Margaret and the family would join me in January 1970.

I did not anticipate needing much clinical earnings on top of my "geographic full-time" salary from the Medical Research Council (MRC), paid through the university, so I did not accept clinical responsibility for kidney patients during the first year or so. I was also writing a nephrology textbook with Henry Gault, called *Nephron Failure*.[52] However, I did agree to follow kidney recipients in the clinic, because only about four to six transplants had been done before I arrived.

Establishing Edmonton's MRC Unit

Encouraged by two leaders in Canadian medicine, Dr. Walter MacKenzie in Alberta and Dr. Malcolm Brown at the MRC in Ottawa, I put together a plan for a MRC Unit in Transplantation Immunology and sent it for consideration to the council in Ottawa. At that time, there were only five or so special MRC research units in Canada, and this would be the first in the field of transplantation immunology. I was to be the co-director with Dr. Erwin Diener, a basic immunologist from Switzerland who had also done research at Sir MacFarlane Burnet's unit in Melbourne, Australia. Local surgeons and others bought into the master plan.

The MRC sent a team to look over the facilities and talk to the people in our group. The impressive team included Dr. Rupert Billingham, a director of the Wistar Institute in Philadelphia who had worked with Dr. Peter Medawar; Dr. Fritz Bach, an experimental immunologist from New York University and later the University of Minneapolis; and Dr. Tony Monaco, an immuno-surgeon from the Deaconess Hospital in Boston.

A month or so later, we were absolutely thrilled when the elaborate plan was accepted by the MRC for immediate funding early in 1970—and generous funding it was, too, lasting until 1982. We received $1- to $2-million annually during that whole time. The unit would provide a bridge between basic immunology (under Diener) and applied clinical transplant immunology (for which I would be responsible). Most of the research carried out between 1970 and 1982 was under the auspices of the MRC Transplant Group.

Tissue types and tissue typing factors

One area of particular interest was estimating the compatibility between donor and recipient tissues—*histocompatibility*—that determines whether they can be grafted effectively. As mentioned previously, in addition to blood types there is another set of factors, attached to the human leukocyte-A system (HLA system) that can determine the severity of the immune response and, in the case of transplantation of organs or tissues, the severity of the rejection of the donor organ or tissues. There are about 60 HLA factors and each individual carries eight: four inherited from his or her mother, and four from his or her father. They are controlled by two genes at each of the four distinct loci on the sixth pair of human chromosomes.[53]

Testing for histocompatibility involves determining the HLA profile of both the donor and recipient and matching them as closely as possible. In the 1960s, tissue typing was not even considered. The field opened up when it was recognized that women who had borne several children develop HLA-factor antibodies in their serum. As explained previously (Chapter 6), this happens when their husbands' HLA-factors migrate from the fetus (which gets its HLA-factors from both mother and father), across the placenta into the mother's body. The mother's immune system sees these factors as foreign and creates antibodies against them. This information proved to be very useful. These women's sera, suitably screened and absorbed, provided an increasingly sophisticated battery of sera for detecting unknown tissue factors on other people, including those whose organs became available for transplantation. From them, tissue typing was born.

In those early days, tissue typing involved isolating the lymphocytes (white cells) from the person who was going to donate an organ and testing them in a typing tray. These trays contained 60 wells, each with a different HLA-factor antibody in it. Donor cells were placed in each well and would either react and be killed by a particular antibody, or be compatible. In this way we could determine the HLA-factors of the donor and know whether they were a match for the organ recipient, who had been previously tested.

Tissue typing was identified as an important area for our research group in Edmonton, and our first venture was to look for understanding of what we assumed—rightly, as it happened—would be a limited number of HLA factors in certain human populations due to geographic isolation and much in-breeding over centuries or millennia. Two such populations were accessible from Edmonton: the Inuit in the Arctic (isolated for about 20 millennia from their Mongolian ancestors by the last Ice Age); and the Hutterites in Alberta (isolated for more than 100 years after being forced to flee Europe because of religious beliefs).

Expeditions to the Arctic

We joined the ongoing research efforts of Dr. Otto Schaeffer of Edmonton and Dr. Jack Hildes of Winnipeg—two well-known physician researchers in Northern medicine—to study the HLA system in the Inuit. We knew that each person carried two out of the possible four gene loci (A, B, C or D) and had eight HLA factors. Within a few years, we knew that locus A had about 20 possible HLA factors, locus B also had 20, locus C had ten and locus D had eight. It was not long before more than 100 factors could be recognized. Matching factors for the A and B genetic loci was important in organ transplantation; matching for region C was shown to be unimportant; and matching for D proved to be the most important—and problematic.

Unlike the HLA factors for loci A, B and C, the HLA-D factors could not be readily identified using the common antibodies in the sera of multiparous women in typing trays (although a few years later we found that this was not really so). Determination of the fourth locus factors— HLA-D—came from research using a different technique: the mixed lymphocyte culture (MLC) test, developed by Fritz Bach and Bernard Amos.[54,55] They found that when cells from different people were mixed in a seven-day culture with cells from another population, they would always stimulate cell division. They then found that they could modify the test by first treating one person's cells with a chemical, mitomycin (Mutamycin), that was normally used to treat some types of cancer. Mitomycin treatment did not kill those cells—they could still stimulate another person's cells to divide in culture—but it made them unresponsive to stimulation by another person's cells in mixed cultures. Thus, if one person's cells were pre-treated with mitomycin, the otherwise bilateral stimulation became a one-way response. The dividing population of cells could now be quantified by their ability to incorporate another chemical, radioactive thymidine, which could be counted in a gamma ray counter. Thus the test became a one-way MLC test.

Working within families, they unexpectedly found that cultures between certain siblings could not mutually stimulate, but each such sibling's cells would always be stimulated by mitomycin-treated cells of both parents and *vice versa*. In other words, a sibling cell that was unable to stimulate another sibling cell would always stimulate both parental cells.

We now know that the facts fit the following model:

Suppose that father has HLA-D x and y factors, and mother HLA-D p and q.

All children HLA-D profiles fall into only one of four categories: D-xp; D-xq; D-yp; or D-yq.

A child with D-xp will stimulate all its siblings and both parents, because it sees at least one different factor, y or q, on each parental cell. But a D-xp child will not stimulate a sibling who is also D-xp. Two such siblings are called HLA-D identical siblings (they are not necessarily twins; nor are fraternal twins necessarily HLA-D identical).

There is a one in four chance that HLA-D status is identical between any two siblings and, using skin grafts between family members, researchers established that these factors were important in transplantation. Later this enabled excellent outcomes for kidney grafts between HLA-D identical siblings.

Of course, it follows that two HLA-D identical siblings will also be *serologically* typed as identical for HLA-A, B and C factors. But if one collects a large panel of *unrelated* people and tests those who appear to be identical for HLA-A, B and C factors (antigens), they will very likely *all* be stimulated to cell division by a mitomycin-treated cell such as D-*xp*.

This finding led to the belief that the one-way mixed lymphocyte test was detecting evidence of an HLA locus that the sera (characterized for their content of antibodies to HLA-A, B and C) were not. It was termed HLA-D.

It was then apparent that the most useful cells for identifying HLA-D would be those that had identical factors at the gene locus, as determined by their reactions in the one-way MLC test. Finding such cells became a priority.

An example of this would be family where the father's HLA-D factors are x and y and the mother's are x and q. Here, both parents share the HLS-D-x factor, by chance.

The children's HLA-D profiles would have to be D-xx, D-xq, D-yx or D-yq.

In this example, cells from a D-xx child, after mitomycin-treatment, are *not able to stimulate either parent*, or some of its siblings. This D-xx is an HLA-D MLC typing cell, in that it is a specific non-stimulator of any other cell that carries HLA D-x.

As the HLA-D factors were identified, there also was confirmation of their importance in predicting graft survival.

To meet the challenges of this research, we needed to find a source of HLA-D typing cells. We looked for a population that likely had a restricted number of HLA factors in their gene pool. It was speculated, correctly, that there would be less diversity of all the HLA factors on the cells of relatively in-bred populations. Such individuals share many genes, including those of the HLA region on chromosome six. With less diversity, there is a greater chance of two parents sharing some of their HLA factors (A, B, C and D) and then producing children with the same HLA-D gene on each of their sixth chromosomes—correctly called homozygous for HLA-D. The one-way MLC test was then used to find the sibling cells that

Figure 7.1 In our research with the Inuit, we visited Inuvik, Tuktoyaktuk and Igloolik in the Arctic.

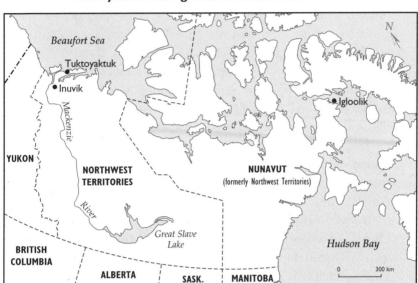

failed to stimulate both parents' cell, establishing that it was homozygous for HLA-D, and therefore a HLA-D typing cell.

Because of their relatively contained gene pool, the Inuit were likely to have a higher proportion of homozygous HLA-D factors. Our aim was to collect these cells, separate them, and circulate them through histocompatibility workshops among the 30 or 40 other laboratories worldwide that were working on the same problem.

Thus, there were two initial objectives to our expeditions to the North:

1) to determine the degree of diversity of Inuit tissue groups with respect to HLA-A, -B, and -C compared with those living in the South (i.e., Edmonton), using our trays loaded with small drops of typing sera (obtained from multiparous women), and

2) to determine if there were cells that could be identified as homozygous HLA-D typing cells. Inuit families tend to be large, so we hoped to find cells that, after Mitomycin exposure, failed to stimulate cell division in cells of both parents when cultured separately with each parent's cells, and could therefore be used to match for HLA-D factors.

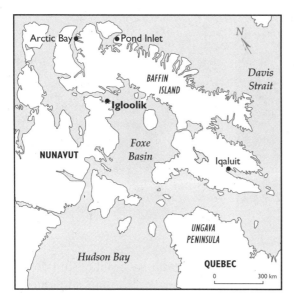

Figure 7.2 The location of the island of Igloolik, in relation to Baffin Island, Ungava Peninsula and Northern Quebec.

We made an initial expedition to Inuvik and Tuktoyaktuk in July 1971 to do ordinary tissue typing of Inuit families (Figure 7.1). This confirmed that the diversity of HLA antigens in this population was very restricted. In June 1972, we went to Igloolik, at the northern end of Hudson Bay (Figure 7.2), to carry out selected skin grafts between those who had previously been tissue-typed to see if we could validly predict altered survival of skin grafts (i.e., prolong survival when the matching was close).

These expeditions were greatly facilitated by Otto Schaeffer, who had practised medicine in the North for ten years or so, could speak several dialects, and was known and trusted by the Inuit. He was also a source of great wisdom about the North and a fascinating person to have as a research colleague. We used him, almost entirely, as our means of obtaining informed consent. Consent was mainly "community consent," although we also asked for individual consent. Schaeffer obtained community consent after meeting with the community elders in various ceremonies and explaining why we wanted their help.

The first trip to Igloolik in the northwestern part of Hudson Bay, not far from the North Pole, involved flying through to Iqaluit (then called Frobisher Bay), capital of Nunavut, and then across Baffin Island to Igloolik. Our expedition consisted of 20 people, including physiologists, anthropologists and our Edmonton group. We arrived at night during the second week of January 1972 to an indescribable cold that I never want to

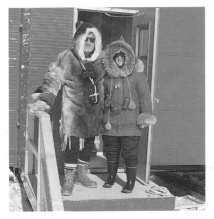 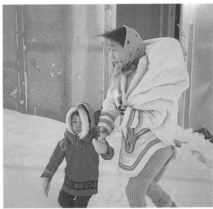

The research team (left) and some of the subjects (right).

experience again! The pilot of the prop-plane did not want to shut down the engines because of the cold, so we had to off-load our equipment, including centrifuges, in the bitter cold of the slip stream from the engines. We worked in the dark, with our only light coming from the headlights of half a dozen skidoos. The wind chill factor must have been -150ºC! We soon warmed up in the natural-gas heated wood and plasterboard buildings set several feet off the ground, in which we were to live for two weeks. During the first week, it was dark all day, everyday, though I recall the sun rising at 12:00 noon on January 12 over the east end of the school roof, then setting at 12:20 p.m. A short day, to be sure, but also a sign of spring.

Our routine was fairly simple. We took blood samples from the population, prepared their white blood cells and sealed them in ampules. The ampules, when prepared and labelled, were thrown out of the front door into a snow bank—our refrigerator. We dug them out and packed them in snow when the time came to leave.

Back in Edmonton, we tissue-typed the population and identified certain cells as good homozygous HLA-D typing cells for MLC tests. We hoped to get a plentiful supply of them for the international workshops,[56] which proved to be more difficult that I had anticipated. We had to travel North again to obtain substantial amounts of blood from those we identified as homozygous for HLA-D.

Putting our laboratory findings to the test

On our third trip to the North in the early summer of 1972, we journeyed back to Igloolik to carry out selective skin-grafting on the people we had tissue-typed in January. We had kept in close contact with the community through Schaeffer, and he agreed to come along to oversee the procedures. Edmonton plastic surgeon, Dr. Mac Alton, carried out the skin grafting. We already knew that the Inuit's HLA diversity was much less than that of outbred populations of the South and, thanks to the tissue typing, we knew the specific HLA factors of the population. We hoped to show that skin grafts between Inuit would last longer than those between members of outbred populations.

Before leaving Edmonton, Alton and I exchanged skin grafts, using auto grafts (grafts of our own skin onto ourselves) as controls, so that we would be able to show what was involved in skin grafting when we arrived at Igloolik. We hoped that showing them what a persistent "take" looked like in comparison to one that had been rejected, and that no harm came to us as a result of the grafts, would make it easier to obtain community agreement to the procedure.

We did not discuss hepatitis B or C viral risks (we knew nothing of HIV at the time) and it was fortunate than none of these viruses were prevalent in the North at that time, otherwise our research would have been disastrous.

We also recruited an experienced nurse who stayed in the community for several months after the procedures to examine the grafts every few days, take photos of the various stages of persistence or graft rejection, and keep a careful log.

The research was successful in showing that skin grafts lasted longer in the Inuit than in Caucasians and that the system could be used to predict the long-term survivors from the short. At the time, it was deemed to be a useful confirmation of the role played by the HLA system in predicting graft survivals. But there was to be a delayed echo from this project.

An unexpected echo of this research

The following is an account of our skin-grafting research as remembered by one of the subjects in the study and reported in *The Globe and Mail*[57] in February 2000. It is disturbing to read that one's research was so poorly understood, and that the subjects could not recall receiving adequate information or giving informed consent.

Several points came to mind as I read Rhoda Katsak's account. She was 15 years old in 1972. The memories I have of these studies is proved false by her account. The graft experiment was not willingly undertaken

In this excerpt from "Sayiyuq: Stories from the Lives of Three Inuit Woman," as reported in *The Globe and Mail*, Rhoda Katsak, who was born 1957, speaks.

I was telling Josh last night about how my scars were itching. They were itching and itching, and it reminded me of the story about how I got them. It was in 1971 or 1972. We were in Igloolik and I was probably about 13 or 14, and this group of scientists, or whoever they were, they came into town. They called themselves anthropologists. I remember it was big deal for these guys to come in. We heard about it before they came. It was like major news in the community, a big study going on in our small town.

The day after they came in, my family was told to go to this building next to the nursing station. That is where they were working, this little building. We went over there, my mother, my brother Jakopie, my older sister Oopah, and myself. I think that my mother had somebody on her back, Ida, maybe, I don't know. I don't know if it was just my family that was tested. I don't think it was everybody in the community, just certain families. They had some sort of a list and I think they were picking names from that list or something. I remember us walking over there.

We did not know what was going on. First they had us climb up and down these three wooden steps, three steps up and three down. We climbed up and down. They wanted to see how much we could do without getting tired.

The big thing I remember though was that they took bits of skin off our forearms. First they made the whole skin area numb, then they took this very long, thin cylinder, like a stick, sharp on one end, and they kind of drilled it into my arm to cut the skin. They took the skin off, it was at the end of this little cylinder thing. It was inside. They did that at three places. Once they took the skin off my arm at three places they put in skin from my sister Oopah and my brother Jake's and mine. I think my mom was there. Of course, we were her children so she had to be there, maybe to consent or something like that. But I don't think it was a matter of her consenting. I don't think she thought of it that way. Then, after they did that, they put bandages on. It did not hurt that much at the time. It hurt later, like a regular cut would, but it did not hurt at all at the time because of the anesthetic….

I remember with my skin grafts they told us that they were trying to find out if a person got burned, if they could get a skin graft from sibling's skin. Maybe they thought Inuk skin was different from Qallunaat skin, I don't know. It sure would have been nice to know what they were doing at the time! Anyways, the grafts did not heal into my skin. Jake's and Oopah's skin fell off and the holes healed over. Those anthropologists are very lucky the cuts weren't on my face....We were told to go back to that place a couple of times because they wanted to check to see if the grafts were staying. We went back, but it was nice to see them go and not stay....I remember being happy when Jake and Oopah's skin fell off my arm. I was happy that I disproved their theory. I have had the scars ever since. They don't go away.

Ethical Dilemma

For medical research on humans, is community consent ever good enough? I had thought it was, and we did our work on that assumption. Later, however, I came to wonder about the validity of it. I now think it was not enough. We should have found a way of explaining it in detail to each graft recipient, and making sure they not only understood what it was about, but also gave individual consent. Relying on the elders was not enough.

Twenty-five years after the fact, I came to realize fully that the consent process for research is of paramount importance for all researchers. The assumption must be made that it is not being fully comprehended prior to participation. Further, consent must be seen as an ongoing process that also includes follow-up responsibility with results and further questions. These three elements—evidence of comprehension, ongoing consent and follow-up responsibility—are still not considered crucially important even in research today, and no attempt is made to ensure or monitor that they take place.

I now believe that funding of research on humans should include these three additional elements in the budget and that funding agencies should not sign off on research projects until evidence is submitted that these elements have been carried out.

by cheerful confident subjects, as we thought. Again, I find that the informed consent process of research—for which I was directly responsible—was inadequate in that subjects (or at least one of them) did not understand what was going on.

The reader will clearly understand why I now question, very seriously, the validity of group consent from community elders—and this was a major element in consent for this research. After we had explained to the elders in their own community meetings, in their own language, there was reason to believe that their promise to explain to the community what they had agreed to was also adequate. But Rhoda's account makes no mention of the fact that the researchers had exchanged skin grafts in just the same way as the research subjects—though these were shown both to the elders and to individual subjects. Nor does she mention that the skin grafts were placed by one of Canada's leading plastic surgeons. There was only minimal risk involved and that diminishes, but by no means abolishes, the need for fully informed consent.

Meanwhile, back in the lab

After these great experiences we were left to consider how much they added to our body of knowledge. At this time, isolated populations all over the world were being tissue-typed and reported, leading to more and more factors being discovered, especially for HLA-A and -B. Although we found several new HLA-D homozygous D-typing cells, we realized that there would always be considerable logistical problems in getting enough of each for use in transplantation work. The provider of these vital cells lived too far away. It was a simple as that.

So we rethought our strategy and decided that a Caucasian isolate population might be more useful in providing homozygous typing cells— which is what the transplant world really needed. Realizing this, our thoughts turned toward the Alberta Hutterites.

Research in Hutterite colonies

Although their restricted breeding customs had only been going on for several hundred years—not thousands, as in the North—all North American Hutterites stem from the limited number of families on the original boat to North America in the 18th century. Further, although many of their descendants had left the colonies, very few, almost nobody, had joined the colonies from the outside world. There had been only 20 to 40 families in the early settlements, so we predicted a limited range of

HLA factors. Also, though marriages between brother and sister were *verboten*, first cousin marriages were frequent. Thus, our hopes were high of finding people whose lymphocytes would act as MLC typing cells (i.e., homozygous for HLA-D factors).

We developed warm relations with the Hutterite colonies. One reason was that they told me I looked like one of them (i.e., bearded, somewhat formal, overweight). In addition, we persuaded the elders that they would be helping the outside community by giving blood. Another reason for our good relations was that we promised to conduct limited health examinations by looking for elevated blood pressure, early diabetes, and a few other easily-screened conditions. They already knew that they had a higher than expected incidence of type-2 diabetes. Further, their use of the University Hospital in Edmonton for any serious illness created another bond. We were also interested in their genealogies, and there is no Hutterite who is not passionately committed to that quest! All in all, we were welcomed at one colony after another until we had tissue-typed all the Dariusleut Hutterite colonies within 120 km (75 miles) of Edmonton—25 colonies in all.

In the 1970s, many of the families had 12 or more children. As anticipated, the HLA factors had restricted expression in comparison to families in the general population. And, to our delight, we found those special cells. Those with these "valuable" cells agreed to give full blood donations on a more or less regular basis, from which we dutifully prepared lymphocytes, froze them in liquid nitrogen (or dry ice) and sent ampules to many major tissue typing centres in the U.S. and Europe. In return we received similar ampules from them.

The technological bombshell

All this activity went on for several years before a technological bombshell burst. It was found that antibodies to HLA-A, -B and -C factors in our tissue typing sera—still mainly derived from healthy multiparous women—could be absorbed by using a mix of blood platelets from a panel of healthy donors. When this was done, some antibodies were left behind. These residual antibodies were then shown to react with HLA-D factors—the factors which, to that point in time, were only detectable by the seven-day mixed MLC test. Since it was becoming increasingly evident that matching for HLA-D factors might be more important than matching for the other factors, this simpler and quicker means of identifying HLA-D was a major breakthrough.

Ethical Dilemma

Did we do the people in these Hutterite communities any real service? Or were we just exploiting their uniqueness for our own purposes? Communication was much better with both the Hutterite elders and individuals than it had been with the Inuit. Care was taken to explain to them why they, as individuals, could help the general community, while also helping their own situation should members later require organ transplantation. In fact, a number of Hutterites did eventually need kidney transplants, usually because of the effects of long-standing high blood pressure and type-2 diabetes in destroying kidneys.

Although indigenous and isolated populations have been much exploited, I believe that our activities with Hutterites were free of harm to those who received us, and, indeed, we could claim— as they would readily admit—to have brought some limited benefits with us, in addition to our needles, syringes and tubes. Further, unlike some isolated groups, they believed in individual consent—though one also needed community consent through their community leaders first. No pressure was ever put on any single individual to participate—as far as I could tell.

We realized we were dealing with a hierarchy of markers on cells: mature red cells have blood group markers (e.g., A, B, O, Rh), blood platelets with HLA-A, B, and C factors (but not HLA-D), and lymphocytes with blood group markers HLA-A, -B, -C and HLA-D.

Overnight, our dependence on our special cells (and those from other laboratories) to determine HLA-D factors disappeared, and with it the *raison d'être* for one of our main research thrusts! *C'est la vie.* We continued to play a role in the rapidly developing field of human histocompatibility research and in Hutterite genetic research,[58] but the special role for Inuit cells had been undermined. The progress of research is ever thus: two steps forward, one step back, and then a step sideways.

Immunologic monitoring

Understanding what was going on in the immune system of those receiving transplants was also rapidly growing. The Edmonton unit's research in that area concerned whether one could serially test for immune reactivity in the circulating lymphocytes or serum to predict when rejection episodes were developing, or, more optimistically, when rejection activity was so low that it warranted decreasing the daily doses of immunosuppressive drugs. We called this immunologic monitoring of the response to the graft.

To do this we needed target cells from the organ *donor*. We obtained these by preparing target lymphocytes from the spleen of the person whose death provided the organ. These cells were separated, purified, placed in vials and deep-frozen in liquid nitrogen. We then tested the transplant *recipient's* serum and lymphocytes against the targets cells of their individual donors

Setting all this up was costly and time-consuming, though we gained a lot of insight. Dr. Calvin Stiller, who was a great stimulus to us during the 18 months he spent in Edmonton, was also committed to the concept of immunological monitoring. After he left to set up a multi-organ transplantation unit in London, Ontario, in 1973, he organized a conference on the topic under the auspices of the Canadian Transplantation Society and invested Dr. Bernie Carpenter from Boston and myself as co-chairs. It was a success and the proceedings were published,[59,60,61] but it also signalled the end of this area of research. We had thought everyone would be obliged to use similar methods to achieve the best transplant survival results. But, as in the histocompatibility research, this did not turn out to be the case; things were evolving elsewhere. Although we could see rejection activity mounting by using these blood parameters, we could also detect it by increasingly sensitive indicators such as blood flow studies of the transplanted kidney or its function, or from microscopic evidence from renal biopsies. In addition, we set up systems to measure the blood levels of various immunosuppressive drugs, especially cyclosporine, which came on the scene in the 1970s.

The cyclosporine era

While I continued to keep things going in tissue typing research, much of my time was also spent looking after patients. I gradually increased my time in following up those who had received transplants, and also took on periods of clinical responsibility on both the renal ward (which eventually had 18 beds) and the in-patient hemodialysis unit (14 beds).

Soon I was facing much the same dilemma as I had at McGill: my research efforts were being diluted by clinical demands, to the point where it was not meeting my own standards, let alone those that might be held by the MRC. This process was accelerated by the departure of

Dr. Mike Higgins in 1978, a nephrologist and director of dialysis. One cannot protect one's research time when there are urgent clinical responsibilities that require attention. I told the MRC, to whom I clearly had a research commitment, and President Pierre Bois understood my predicament and was not opposed to this use of my time. Still, it was the beginning of the end of the research group funding.

One of the last big clinical research thrusts was the clinical trial of cyclosporine (Neoral or Sandimmune) in Canada, organized mainly through Dr. Stiller's group. I also played an organizing role in this and it took quite a lot of planning time. At the time, the Canadian trial was considered one of the premier studies in North America and, in 1983, was published in the prestigious *New England Journal of Medicine*.[62]

Overview of the science of transplantation

In retrospect, I am astounded by the progression of transplantation science since those early experiments with the twin girls in Montreal in 1958 to my work in immunology, which ended in 1982. Nowhere are the advances in medical sciences during the last 60 years more visible and dramatic than in the evolution of organ transplantation.

Figure 7.3, transplant of the organ, shows the five main thrusts of new knowledge that converged to make transplantation possible and successful.

These main thrusts in the evolution of organ transplantation are:

1. **Pathophysiology of disease**
    Several branches of medical science contribute to the understanding of disease, its localization to one or diffusion to several organs, its physiological disturbances of function and distortion of structure (pathology) and finally measures that support the person up to the day of surgery, even though a vital organ has failed (e.g., dialysis).

2. **Transplantation immunology**
    Of premier importance to the success of transplantation is the nature of the immune response, including the role of lymphocytes, the immunology of disease and of rejection, the factors involved in tissue foreignness and tissue matching, and the whole subject of immunosuppression.

Figure 7.3 Transplant of an organ.

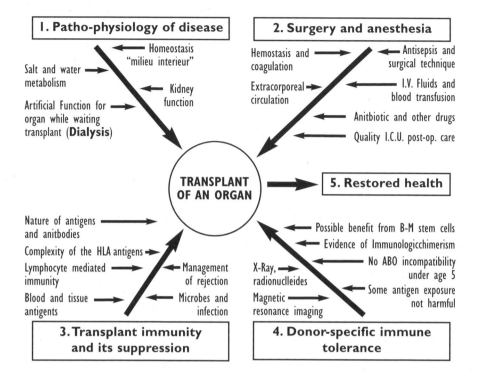

3. **Tolerance induction**

   I have given prominence to specific immune tolerance induction because I predict that discoveries in the next ten years will make this the main thrust in managing immune response in transplantation, though we are not at this point yet. My personal reminiscences on this area have recently been published.[63]

4. **Surgery**

   Several branches of medical science have enabled modern surgery to become the technical marvel that it is today. Included in this is the understanding of infection and the importance of antisepsis and maintenance of bacterial sterility, the whole history of anesthesia, the restoration of body fluids to normal, in volume and composition (homeostasis), the maintenance of normal coagulability in the blood (hemostasis), and the ability to place an organ on systems for extra-corporeal circulation (e.g., keeping the rest of the body functioning during bypass surgery when the diseased heart is operated on or replaced). All these aspects allow surgeons to do increasingly incredible procedures.

5. **Restored health through post-operative care**
The medical sciences that are used to manage patients after transplantation include the treatment of rejection and infection, and the monitoring of transplanted organ function by means of various forms of imaging.

Most of these areas of knowledge have origins that date to the Renaissance, but their real flowering and convergence has occurred in the last 60 years. Organ transplantation was initially brought to reality by means of the kidney, but then expanded to include heart, heart-lung, liver, pancreas, small bowel, and limb transplants.

The research done in the Edmonton MRC transplantation unit contributed to this evolution in medical science. Indeed, from 1971 to 1982, our members published more than 300 papers in the scientific literature on various basic and clinical aspects of transplantation.

Ironically, the most significant success in our group began in the field of transplantation, but culminated in a breakthrough in another area entirely.

A scientific gem, mined in Edmonton

The development of transplant work in Edmonton is a tale of achievement that is the stuff of romance, courage and determination that has been deservedly rewarded by success and scientific recognition. It concerns tiny groups of cells in the pancreas called the islets of Langerhans.

The prime mover for all this research is Ray Rajotte, PhD, who is now the director of the Surgical-Medical Research Institute at the University of Alberta. His story is worth relating as a paradigm for what research is all about. (Because he is not a medical doctor, the clinicians involved in the project often get most of the limelight, but that does not worry Rajotte. He is a scientist: a cryobiologist, immunologist, and cell and tissue preservationist.)

Rajotte started off as a radiology technician in Edmonton but, not being satisfied with that, he spent his spare time and summer vacations working with surgeons at the Royal Alexandra Hospital in pursuit of aspects of transplantation. In 1971, he developed a keen interest in preserving tissues by first permeating the tissue with a cryoprotective agent, dimethylsulfoxide (DMSO), then freezing them in liquid nitrogen to sub-zero temperatures. The tissue, stored at -196 °C, was then re-warmed using microwave energy. He was successful in recovering activity in frozen fully-differentiated fetal mouse hearts in our unit[64]—no mean achievement—but had no real success in recovering frozen organs that required the blood supply to be reconnected when implanting.[65] The functioning cells of an organ might survive, but the capillaries, necessary for ongoing survival, did not.

He then moved to the preservation of the islets of Langerhans, that part of the pancreas that secretes insulin and other hormones. Working in association with the transplantation service, he perfected ways of preparing pancreatic islets from the pancreas of cadaveric organ donors. Islets do not need an independent blood supply; they can live by simple diffusion with the fluid space known as the extra-cellular space. Clinical studies were pursued for the next 25 years, with varying success, until he and his team achieved the breakthrough that all research scientists crave.[66] This was recognized by a standing ovation when the work was presented to the American Society of Transplantation at Chicago in May 2000—only the second time of which I am aware that scientists gave a colleague such an ovation. This long period of research resulted in publication in the *New England Journal of Medicine*,[67] which gave him the privilege of online pre-publication in recognition of the importance of the discovery.

What they had shown by using what is now known as the Edmonton protocol is simply this: patients with severe type-1 diabetes—also known as juvenile diabetes—could be cured. The process involves first obtaining pancreas tissue from cadaver donors, separating out the islets of Langerhans and preserving the islets until there are enough to treat a recipient. Patients are put on a special combination of immunosuppressive medications in the post-transplant period. The suspension of islet tissue is then infused into the portal vein (the large vein taking blood from the intestines back through the liver). When given in this manner, the islets lodge in the liver, and live and function there as if they were in a pancreas, secreting insulin in proportion to the dictates of the blood sugar level, as is normal.

This exciting train of research started in the MRC transplantation group in the early 1970s, and I had the privilege of being the supervisor of both Rajotte's master's thesis, and co-supervisor (with Dr. Geoffrey Voss) of his subsequent doctorate work. But it was the work of Rajotte and his colleague that stunned the world of diabetes in 2000.

The fundamental sciences upon which medicine depends have been greatly extended. The laboratory has come to furnish alike to the physician and to the surgeon a new means for diagnosing and combating disease. The education of the medical practitioner under these changed conditions makes entirely different demands in respect to both preliminary and professional training.

For twenty-five years past there has been an enormous over production of uneducated and ill trained medical practitioners. This has been in absolute disregard of the public welfare and without any serious thought of the interests of the public. Taking the United States as a whole, physicians are four or five times as numerous in proportion to population as in older countries like Germany. In view of these facts, progress for the future would seem to require a very much smaller number of medical schools, better equipped and better conducted than our schools now, as a rule, are.

A hospital under complete educational control is as necessary to a medical school as is a laboratory of chemistry or pathology. High grade teaching within a hospital introduces a most wholesome and beneficial influence into its routine. Trustees of hospitals, public and private, should therefore go to the limit of their authority in opening hospital wards to teaching, provided only that the universities secure sufficient funds, on their side, to employ as teachers men who are devoted to clinical science.

Any state of the Union or any province of Canada is better off without a medical school than with one conducted in a commercial spirit and below a reasonable plane of efficiency. Our hope is that this report will make plain, once and for all, that the day of the commercial medical school has passed.

Medical Education in the US and Canada
Abraham Flexner, 1910

8

Academic medicine: Perils and pleasures

ACADEMIC MEDICINE WAS RESHAPED by Abraham Flexner's report on medical education to the Carnegie Foundation for the Advancement of Teaching in 1910.[68] As a result of this report, many inadequate and sub-standard. North American "degree mills" were closed; standards were set for pre-medical education; and it was deemed that medical faculty should be full-time and committed to doing research, which meant that regular medical practitioners were largely excluded from teaching in medical schools (this has since changed somewhat). These changes were not acceptable to the great educator and clinician, Sir William Osler, who wrote: "I cannot imagine anything more subversive to the highest ideal of the clinical school than to hand over our young men, who are to be our best practitioners, to a group of teachers who are *ex officio* out of touch with the conditions under which these young men will live."[69]

Nevertheless, Flexner set the template for the 20th century academic medical faculty. The significance of medical faculties as the focal point of clinical research was further boosted, particularly after World War II, by the explosion of knowledge of the mechanisms of disease and the enormous increase in funds available for research.

What this created, in essence, was academic medicine: the notion that medical education should be comprised of a sound knowledge of the medical sciences, the methodology of research, as well as the mechanisms of disease and the scientific basis of therapies. The unique aspect of, and fascination with, academic medicine is the privilege it affords the individual of having several irons in the fire, aside from the main research focus. Thus, the academic physician is part laboratory researcher, part clinical investigator, part clinician to patients, part teacher to students and residents, and part administrator. Unfortunately, sometimes these roles conflict, resulting in ethical dilemmas.

I. Continuity of care

As with most physicians in academic circles, I would take periodic clinical responsibilities for individuals. We called these periods "stints," as if one could assume people's illnesses just like that, run with them for two weeks, or a month, and then pass them on to someone else. Personally, I have never been able to adjust fully to this rotation of clinical responsibility for individuals. It seems to put one's own interests—in my case, the other demands on my time—before those of the patients one serves. The net loss is continuity of care. Each new clinician—and inevitably in this sort of system there will be several—is essentially starting from scratch, albeit armed with the chart and other documentation. It is time-consuming for the clinician, frustrating for the patient who must repeat his or her story *ad nauseam* and compromises the quality and continuity of care. I view this system as an affront to professional ethics.

This fragmented responsibility has become accepted practice in the last 20 years, not only for those in academic medicine, but throughout the profession. Even in such places as the intensive care unit (ICU) where individuals are cared for only through short, severe phases of an illness, the same phenomenon is rife. I recall discussing the moral distress of ICU residents with my ethics colleague, Dr. Paul Byrne, in the 1990s. The residents had complained to us during ethics consultations that the attending staff physicians were on the unit for such short periods—often just seven days—and that their ability to make informed decisions was limited. During their first two days, they were paralysed by their insufficient knowledge of complex situations, and during the last two days they did not want to compromise their successor's decision-making freedom. In effect, they were in full command of decision-making only during the middle three days. It is incredible, yet widely so in various ICU settings. Of course, this would not apply to new admissions, such as those who were admitted on their first day of ICU duty.

In the past, the anchor person for a ward was the resident physician or surgeon, who was on duty more or less continuously, which was a serious problem for that individual's physical and mental health, but at least one knew everything that was going on with one's patients. One of my moments of pride, long ago as a house-physician at St. Bartholomew's Hospital, was when the chief said to a patient: "I guess you can be discharged home now! Does that please you?" He replied: "Sure Doc, provided that Dr. Dossetor agrees that I am ready to go." That remark did a lot for my ego, though I am not sure that the snort emitted by the chief was that fruitful for my reputation! Nowadays, the continuity provided by the resident physicians is gone. No one works more than two nights without one night off, and there is a lot of cross-covering among services, so that a resident might admit patients to several different services during one night. He or she then leaves the day staff to pick up the traces and read the progress notes. That is not optimal continuity of care—which should be one of the benefits of being in hospital—but it may be the best that can be, given the staffing stresses that beset universal health care insurance systems.

Despite my misgivings about this lack of continuity, I went along with the system at the University of Alberta simply because that was the way things were done. Fortunately, in nephrology we were able to mitigate this conflict by introducing two new programs to ensure continuity of care: the "nephrology nurse clinician" program and a dedicated, "long-term nephrologist" concept.

The Nephrology Nurse Clinician (NNC) program came about after an incident where we called a patient in for a kidney transplant thinking that she was in good shape for surgery, only to find that no one knew that she had a valid medical reason why she should not be operated upon right then. One of the senior nurses said to me, "You guys really do not know these dialysis patients well enough. I believe you should do something about getting to know them better." She was dead right. We developed the NNC program, where selected renal nurses received special training in nephrology and functioned as more or less permanent fixtures on the physician-care team. They turned out to be terrific in that role and greatly improved continuity of care.

We also introduced a program whereby each patient had his or her own long-term nephrologist, in addition to whichever physician was on daily call for short periods in rotation. The long-term physician became involved in every decision with long-term implications. Although this helped mitigate some of the difficulties, the underlying problem remained. As it becomes progressively more specialized, modern medicine has distanced physicians from those they serve and, as a consequence, care has become more fragmented.

2. Double dipping

In taking on clinical responsibilities, the person in academic medicine also faces a potential conflict of interest in regard to payment. As a career investigator of the MRC to do research, a person is paid a salary from public funds more or less on a full-time basis. But at the same time, the person is also able to bill on a fee-for-services basis as a physician by undertaking clinical practice. Some would say this provides an opportunity for double dipping into the public purse.

One solution would be for all physicians to be on salary from the government—such as occurs in Sweden, and as used to be the case in the U.K. But others foresee that the introduction of fully-salaried academic physicians might lead to a profound hemorrhage of Canadian academic physicians to the U.S..

3. Clinician and recruiter of subjects for research

Another ethical dilemma inherent in the multiple roles in academic medicine is the fact that, as a clinical researcher, I was responsible for both a clinical research trial of cyclosporine and for recruiting subjects, some of whom were my patients. It was important to my career that I enrol as many patients as possible; the larger the patient sample in my study, the more pertinent the end results. But at the same time I was personal physician to some of those who entered the trial as research subjects. This investigator/responsible physician duality creates a serious conflict of interest. We had no sound scientifically valid evidence that this drug would work better than the existing immunosuppressive regimen, and because we were not conducting a blinded controlled trial, we knew whether our patients were getting the old or new therapy. In effect we were asking the patients to trust our opinion that this was a significant therapeutic advance, even though it had never been proven in kidney transplant recipients.

4. The profit motive

In recent years, the funding sources of medical research have gradually changed. No longer are the main funding agents the government (using tax dollars) or the philanthropic institutions. Now, the pharmaceutical industry, sometimes in conjunction with government, is the main funding source. Previously there was accountability to the public through the funding agents' scientific peer-review panels that reviewed progress at the end of each granting period when more funds were requested. Now researchers are accountable to the profit-driven pharmaceutical industry.

Increasingly, the interests of medical researchers have become allied to the interests of the drug industry. To obtain funding, research clinicians are now obliged to side with these private interests, finding new treatments for certain widespread—hence potentially profitable—conditions in the developed world (e.g., obesity, depression), but not necessarily for more serious conditions, such as malaria or HIV/AIDS, in the developing world. Should we not be considering the research needs of sick people (the populations that research should serve) as well as the profit-driven agendas of industry and its stockholders, the new funders of clinical research? It used to be that the clinical researcher could focus on the former and have no concerns about the latter, but this is no longer the case.

In the best of all possible worlds, the interests of industry and those of patients coincide, as was the case in the Canadian cylosporine clinical trials in the mid-1980s, which was funded by both the MRC and Sandoz (now Novartis). Problems arise when the best interests of industry and patient do not mesh, such as the following two cases illustrate.

AIDS RESEARCH

Question: Why is so much more AIDS research directed at developing new treatments than into vaccines that might mitigate the spread of this disease, particularly in its new epidemic forms in sub-Saharan Africa, for example, and elsewhere in the developing world?

Answer: A vaccine that eliminates HIV infection would confer great benefit to people but generate less profit to those who produce it than new drugs that prolong life but do not cure the affliction.

IMMUNE RESEARCH

Question: Why is so much more money spent on developing new and better drugs for controlling the immune response to a transplant than is spent on the holy grail of transplantation—the induction of donor-specific immunologic tolerance?

Answer: Donor-specific immunologic tolerance would lead to much less use of immunosuppressive drugs, and eventual withdrawal from dependence on these drugs. Those who develop the drugs profit by continued dependence on them.

It is small wonder that these conflicts of interest have become an ethical trap in academic medical research at the clinical and basic level. Small wonder, too, that the need has grown over the years for greater probing by the research ethics review process of proposals for clinical research, not only into informed consent, potentially vulnerable research subjects and the like, but also into the motivation and integrity of investigators to perform this type of research.

The difficulties inherent in this relationship between a researcher and industrial funder is aptly illustrated in the Dr. Nancy Olivieri case,[70] a veritable ethical quagmire, with ingredients including:

- an investigator with originality and drive, in search of something new for a fatal condition;
- a drug company that saw an opportunity to make a fortune;
- a gag clause in the researcher's contract that safeguarded the company's interest if the research results were not as positive as expected;
- an investigator who signed the gag clause without disclosing this to the hospital administrator or the Research Ethics Board;
- poor clinical results in the research that impelled public disclosure by the investigator; leading to threats of a legal suit by the drug company;
- appeals in vain, by the investigator, for support from the hospital and the university;
- two arbitration efforts by outsiders;
- accusation of conflict of interest between one of these outside assessors and the drug company.

This case is the subject of a chapter in a book about the relationship between the pharmaceutical world and physician investigators, and it may not, yet, be the end of the story.[71] I refrain completely from trying to assess the case or making any judgement—though my natural sympathy is with the investigator—but it is worth considering the ingredients.

Outside of the research environment, the same conflict of interests may affect the specialist's and family physician's office practice—in particular their prescribing practices. Physician integrity may be compromised[72] (or seen to be compromised) by marketing strategies such as:

- free entertainment of physicians by drug firms with everything from pizza lunches at hospital functions to trips to Acapulco;

- subtle influences at pharmaceutical company-funded opportunities for continued medical education;
- sophisticated presentations of the latest therapeutic advances by well-trained pharmaceutical company representatives (detailers) during regular visits to doctor's offices;
- collection of an individual physician's prescribing habits from pharmacy information, that are then sold to the pharmaceutical industry to provide data that are used by drug reps to target the physician;
- payment to the physician for enrolling patients in so-called phase 4 marketing trials of new medications.[73]

I experienced this difficult field of industry-physician interaction first-hand when I agreed to be a consultant to a well-known manufacturer of artificial kidneys and dialyzing membranes. The warmth of their invitation was leavened by the fact that the medical director was an old friend from my days at McGill. For two successive years, my wife and I were invited to meet with the rest of the Canadian nephrologist consultants and the company people: the first year in Nassau, Bahamas, and the second year in Acapulco, Mexico. I realized that my integrity was compromised when the University of Alberta Hospital Purchasing Department, in Edmonton, asked me for my recommendation on equipment for the dialysis unit. They were prepared to spend close to one million a year and had quotes from several suppliers including, of course, the firm for whom I was a consultant. I, together with two others, had to recommend one of them. I promptly resigned from the consultancy even though I genuinely thought that the supplier to whom I had been consultant was the best.

5. Academic privileges

Academic members of professional medical societies have many occasions to travel to medical/clinical-research meetings. Sometimes these trips are charged to research grants, or to pools of departmental travel funds, or, increasingly, to the organization, such as a pharmaceutical company, that is sponsoring the conference or talk. Two medical meetings are acceptable as tax-deductible professional educational experiences each year, which is fair enough. However, in my case, I was out of town about once a month for most of the 20 years between 1965 and 1985, often to present a paper, occasionally just to be there and sometimes to lecture. In all, I took about 250 trips.

Before 1986, when my interest in medical ethics blossomed, I attended more or less regularly 13 society meetings, including the International Transplant Society, the Canadian Society of Transplantation, the American Society of Nephrology, the Canadian Society of Nephrology, the International Society of Nephrology, the Royal College of Physicians and Surgeons (Canada), the Society of Artificial Internal Organs, the European Dialysis and Transplant Association, the Canadian Society of Clinical Investigation, the American Society Histocompatibility, the U.S. Society of Clinical Investigation, the American College of Physicians, and the Western Association of Physicians. Two of these annual meetings took place in Australia, others were held in Stockholm, Paris, New York, Helsinki, Florence, Athens, Denmark, the U.K., Los Angeles and Jerusalem. And this is not the whole list.

In addition to all those meetings, I also travelled as a member of two peer-review panels to review research grants for the MRC and the Kidney Foundation of Canada I co-founded—see Chapter 5. Then there was a three-year stint as an examiner in internal medicine for the Royal College of Physicians and Surgeons when I travelled to Montreal, Toronto and Vancouver to meet candidates.

Last, I was invited to give talks at different places as a visiting professor. Under this rubric I was privileged to tour South Africa, visit transplant units in Poland and France, make two trips to Germany, and a number of trips to India (see Chapter 9), as well as many such trips within Canada. For these, travel expenses were paid by the inviting organization.

This amount of travel sounds excessive, I know. I sometimes wonder if it was all necessary. As I go through some of the occasions in my mind I try to recall how valuable these trips were, keeping in mind that they were all indirectly funded—but often in full—by the taxpayer. I wonder which of these meetings I would have gone to if I had had to pay for the trips out of my own pocket. These thoughts lead to several crucial questions:

- Would one's research have been slower and of lesser impact without these personal interactions?
- Would one's patients have been worse off without them?

The answers to both questions are affirmative, though it would be impossible to provide tangible proof. These meetings and personal interactions allow someone in academic medicine to increase his or her knowledge, to test out ideas and to discover what others with similar aspirations are thinking. In my opinion, this has an impact on how one would advise patients on their problems and treatment. It is hard to be more definitive, which is why this remains one of the ethical dilemmas facing those in academic medicine.

6. Relationships in research

In research there are several kinds of relationship, each with its own ethical implications. There are, of course, the relationships with one's colleagues (other investigators, research fellows, graduate students, trainee residents) and relationships with research subjects.

Subjects in research do not share the doctor-patient relationship in the same way as those who come to a physician for treatment and advice on their problems. In the research setting, they become *subjects* (no longer *patients*) and the ethical question centres on the validity of the researcher's methods in his or her quest to advance the field by obtaining new generalizable knowledge. At the same time, the clinical researcher may, in fact, still be the principal advisor on the person's individual patient problems. No one has really resolved this dilemma, except to keep emphasizing the importance of recognizing and acknowledging its duality.

While much attention has been paid to the relationship with subjects, little has focused on relationships with colleagues in research, yet this too is an important area of research ethics. The researcher is often faced with decisions about the priorities of ideas (especially when the idea came from a junior colleague), the degree of actual participation in the research (especially senior research colleagues who may have contributed nothing more than acquisition of research funds), the recruitment of research subjects, and the assessment of results and the writing of manuscripts. All these aspects need honest recognition and balance if integrity is to be maintained. Usually there is consensus, though the scientific world has many tales where the process became tarnished by jealousy, injustice, plagiarism, conflict of interest and even fraud. It is in such areas that research often creates ethical hazards for researchers.

The limits of teaching

Although the teaching component of one's duties in academic medicine does not necessarily present ethical dilemmas, it is worth commenting on its inherent limitations. One might expect that teaching would be a point where the life of academic medicine is most vibrant. Unfortunately, I do not believe that is the case. Classes of 115 students make teaching a distant process where interaction with individuals is confined to short periods of conversation before or after the lecture or demonstrations. Teaching on the ward or at the bedside, although a fascinating experience for physicians and one that I treasure, does not lend itself to forging real relationships. I remember more such episodes when I was being taught than when I was teaching—probably because of the one-on-one tutorial system used at Oxford and the teaching rounds at Bart's for medical students. Aside from those experiences, the teaching process does not generate, for me, a wealth of positive memories. I regret this, but have to acknowledge it as a fact.

My most engaging experiences as a teacher were with graduate students taking masters or doctorate degrees, or graduate trainees doing research fellowships, and more prolonged encounters with trainee residents on the wards in internal medicine, nephrology or transplantation immunology. Supervising graduate students' work is one of the true privileges of academic life. Through the years, I was involved with more than 35 people in this category, and they have greatly enriched my academic life.* A supervisor of graduate students needs to be genuinely interested in two things: the selected area of the graduate's research, and the master's or doctoral candidate him- or herself. It is easy to give students short shrift because they are fairly isolated, though dedicated, individuals who do not have strong representation in the halls of academia. One must take care not to overly ration one's time for them.

When all is said and done, the life that I experienced in academic medicine, with its triad of medical science research, teaching and the care of patients, was all I could have dreamed of or hoped for. I believe, also, that I was privileged to have this exposure at a time when there were enormous medical advances. My life was enriched by this growth of

* I wish to acknowledge my debt to those I supervised: at McGill, Yosh Taguchi, Jack Oh, Dana Zborowski, Helen Gorman, Doug Ackman, Bernard Koch, J. Knackstedt, Ralph Bilefsky, P. Rege, R.C. Lohmann, H.C. Rudwal, Stan Lannon and Basab Mookerjee; and in Alberta, Leslie Olsen, Molly Johnny, Kelvin Bettcher, Ray Rajotte, Locksley McGann, Basab Mookerjee, Ted Kovithavongs, Gilles Leclair, Sue Saidman, Marek Jacobisiak, R. Sharma, Chakko Jacob, Peter McConnachie, Joy Haystead (Schlaut), Vincent Lao, Linda Hyschka (Marchuk), Donna Hoopfner, Quim Madrenas, Larry Wiser, Anita Molzahn, Tricia Marck, Donna Wilson and Tim Lambert.

knowledge in all areas. Will it be so for the next generation of medical academics? I believe so, even though there are hazards that one can already see: more detachment, greater dependency on computer-generated knowledge and less capability to cover the waterfront of accumulating knowledge, to name but a few.

I saw, indeed, the conception needed before me but I could not grasp it and give it expression. While in this mental condition I had to undertake a longish journey on the river. Lost in thought I sat on the deck of the barge, struggling to find the elementary and universal conception of the ethical which I had not discovered in any philosophy.

Sheet after sheet I covered with disconnected sentences, merely to keep myself concentrated on the problem. Late on the third day, at the very moment when, at sunset, we were making our way through a herd of hippopotamuses, there flashed on my mind, unforeseen and unsought, the phrase "Reverence for Life."

The iron door had yielded; the path in the thicket had become visible. Now I had found my way to the idea in which affirmation of the world and ethics are contained side by side! Now I knew that the ethical acceptance of the world and of life, together with the ideals of civilization contained in this concept, has a foundation in thought.

—Albert Schweitzer, 1915
Lambaréné Hospital, Gabon, West Africa[74]

9

Ethics in the developing world: India

AT THIS JUNCTURE, I WILL STEP BACK for a moment to reflect on the evolution of medical and clinical science and medical ethics in a broader international context. As my experiences in nephrology and research were unfolding, I was also informed by a series of professional visits to my birthplace, India. There, I had the opportunity to contrast my Western experience with the realities of the developing world, albeit in one of the more prosperous of those nations.

I am left wondering what the right interplay is between reductionist science, the replacement of diseased organs in a few sick individuals, and the broad human dilemmas—poverty, ignorance, and unmitigated deprivation—in Canada and in the developing world. Is there an inevitable erosion of what Albert Schweitzer calls reverence for life? This dynamic dialectic has no clear answer, and yet it is critically important for our global civilization.

Certainly, there is a harsh contrast between the Western and Indian approaches to the delivery of health care. Allocation of resources takes on new meaning in the developing world, where the contrast between care available for those with private incomes and the vast bulk of the impoverished population is before one's eyes—though, sadly, one learns to ignore it. I also witnessed an awakening of bioethics in the Indian health delivery environment that differed with bioethics in the West. Of course, ethics in general has existed in Eastern Societies through the millennia, though usually the systems are strongly based on the ethical precepts of different religious faiths. All faiths, however, have the Golden Rule in some form or other: "Do unto others as you would have them do unto you." In contrast to ethics in the West, I did not become aware of any secular ethics in India, except those that are based on Western concepts.

CONTEMPORARY INDIAN POLITICS

When the Indian Congress political party was founded in 1885, its members proposed economic reforms and a larger role in the formation of British policy for India. In 1920, the Congress began a campaign of passive resistance, led by Mohandas Karamchand Gandhi, against restrictions on the press and political activities. The Congress party was divided on approaches to economic reform; the conservatives favoured cautious reform whereas the leftists, led by Jawaharlal Nehru, urged socialism.

At the outbreak of World War II, the Congress voted for neutrality but when India came under Japanese attack it agreed to co-operate in the war effort in exchange for post-war reforms toward a democratic government. Britain gave India its independence in 1948. Jawaharlal Nehru (1889–1964), the leader of the Congress Party, reluctantly accepted the partition of the Indian subcontinent and the formation of the state of Pakistan. Gandhi was murdered by a Hindu fanatic the same year. Partition gave recognition to the deep antipathy that Muslims feel towards Hindus—though Hinduism is more tolerant of this difference.

After partition, the Congress, as the largest party, governed India under Nehru's leadership. After Nehru's death, his daughter, Indira Gandhi, became prime minister in 1966. In the 1971 national elections and the 1972 state elections, Indira's faction won solid victories, but in a reaction to her emergency rule, it lost the election of 1977. After her assassination in 1984, her son Rajiv Gandhi succeeded to the leadership. Although he led the Congress to re-election in 1984, the party was defeated in 1989 because of scandals and became the major opposition party.

Following Rajiv's assassination during the 1991 election campaign, P.V. Rao became head of the Congress party, and prime minister later that year. In 1996, scandal again led voters to reject Congress at the polls, and the leadership passed in 1998 to Rajiv Gandhi's Italian-born widow, Sonia Gandhi, a political newcomer. The Congress party did poorly, however, in the late 1999 elections and the ruling party became the conservative Hindu BJP (Bharatiya Janata Party), led by Atal Behari Vajpayee. In May 2004, the Congress Party regained power and as leader of the party, Sonia Gandhi was expected to become prime minister. However, she declined the position in favour of Manmohan Singh.

I spent my early years in India and have returned several times after being shipped off to boarding school in England. My parents moved back to the U.K. in 1938, but 15 years later I returned to India to serve as a medical officer with the Brigade of Ghurkhas. Presumably as a result of these early bonds, I have taken every opportunity to journey to India; since 1974, I have made eight visits.

In recounting some of these trips, I have included some details (see sidebar for political context) so that readers can appreciate what it was like to be a medical consultant visitor in India, and also glean the scope of the ethical dilemmas. I have tried to capture the medical ethos of my hosts and to build up the contrast with practices in Canada. Ethics is embedded in relationships; therefore, one must know the context to appreciate the ethical aspects of a professional experience.

December 1974

I was invited to give several talks at the Congress of the Indian Medical Association in Calcutta, and then to visit the kidney centre at Vellore, in Tamil Nadhu, in south central India. Dr. A.B. Mukerjee, the Chief of Medicine, who had arranged for my participation at the Congress, met me at Calcutta airport on December 23. To my surprise, I was able to forgo customs and immigration formalities as Mukerjee had taken care of it all; one of the senior officials had been his patient! Within five minutes we were adrift in the sea of bullock carts, dhoti-clad figures, ancient buses, wandering cows and dogs, inhaling the curiously nostalgic smell of jute and burnt cow dung. All the sensory memories from 21 years earlier came flooding back.

Mukerjee and I dined in my spacious room at the Calcutta Medical Research Institute and chatted about his nephrology protégée in Edmonton, Dr. Mrinal Dasgupta, whom they wanted to attract back to his alma mater. I suspected, in fact, that that was the unstated reason for my invitation to Calcutta.

The next morning, I woke to the sounds of the city drifting to my tenth floor window as it gradually came to life: bicycle bells, car horns, hooters of every type, motor and truck engines, hammering and knocking. At 10:45 I was asked to see a five-year-old patient of Mukerjee's, who had Hodgkin's lymphoma and nephrotic syndrome. He had been treated expertly with prednisone and cyclophosphamide (Cytoxan or Neosar) and was in complete remission. I made what contribution I could to this well-managed case, but there was nothing much to say except to admire and approve what had already been done.

At 11:30, after ten minutes of technological struggle (wrong voltage, fusing things, etc.), I began my talk to the staff on the management of chronic renal failure, with pauses while the projector thought things over. We then enjoyed a curry luncheon in the guest suite with five or six physicians, where renal cases were discussed. Calcutta was seeking to develop a policy for chronic renal failure—a daunting enough task for countries in the affluent West, an almost incredible task for India—which is why they hoped to lure Dasgupta back.

The opening ceremony to the Indian Medical Association was held in a vast marquee erected on the Maidan, a large open area in the middle of Calcutta. Long speeches were made—all in English—mostly concerning the problems of the medical profession and government in Bengal. Government-salaried MDs are not paid enough, so the state is chronically short of doctors. There was no discussion of doctor's fees or fee schedules because 75 per cent of these MDs are in private practice and charge what they will. But there was a great deal of discussion about the need for more government support of the pharmaceutical industry, which was in a bad way because high taxes had driven out the European and U.S. firms, and local companies could not make enough drugs of adequate quality, and were also taxed. I will not go into the question of patents and the breaking of them—a commonplace practice in India.

The last part of Christmas Eve was spent having dinner at the Calcutta Club, a faded remnant of the grandeur of the Raj. The large cool lounges with enormously high ceilings were festooned with Christmas decorations, tastefully placed between the trophy heads, mounted weapons and portraits on the walls. Dozens of turbaned bearers, dressed all in white, whisked around the lounging members. Of the hundred or so people there, only three were white. I felt very privileged.

On Christmas day, I attended the whitewashed St. Paul's Cathedral, which is sheltered by large shady trees and circled by well-kept lawns. From the outside, it had an old Raj look about it, but inside it was alive and packed with Indian people (even though less than one per cent of the 900 million Indian citizens are Christian). I was moved as the sun streamed in the Gothic diamond-patterned windows. Sparrows flitted about in the rafters under the tall roof, 18 metres (60 feet) or so above our heads, and seemed to go into a crescendo of twittering after the organ's final chords of "Christ was born in Bethlehem" died out. The main effort of this church was to help the children of those who live in the street slums of Calcutta, the bustees as they are called.

That afternoon, back at the medical congress, I was whisked onto the platform, given a rose buttonhole and festooned with a four-foot garland of jasmine interspersed with red roses. I listened to a half-dozen speeches about the state of medicine in Bengal and in India in general. I became alert very smartly, when the Chair asked for a few words from the "leader of the Canadian delegation." As there were only two white faces in this assembly of 4,000 physicians—mine and the leader of the Australian delegation—I realized the Chair was referring to me, so I gave an impromptu speech conveying greetings and best wishes from the president and board of the Canadian Medical Association (CMA) to the delegates at the Golden Jubilee Congress of the Indian Medical Association. This seemed to cover things alright, which was just as well because I am certain the CMA had no idea it had a delegation there, any more than I had any idea of who was the current CMA president.

My only critical comment of the Congress is that it was too long on speeches, and too short on medicine. Murray Clarke's talk on burns and their prevention was preceded by a 25-minute speech by the head of the Medical Council of India and a 20-minute speech by the vice-chancellor of a university on the importance of medical progress in modern India or some such fatuity.

Perhaps these interminable introductions are the reason everyone is always late. On December 26, I was due to speak at 9:00 a.m. At 9:03, I was still waiting outside the Calcutta Hospital for transportation to the SSK PGI (about ten minutes' drive). In a panic I decided to go independently by cab to the hospital, then rushed across the hospital ground, ran up three floors in the pathology building, along the veranda, past several lolling delegates and into the lecture hall at exactly 9:15. Only one man was there! Yes, it was the right place. Yes, it was the right time. Yes, everything was under control and starting shortly. By 9:30 there were 150 people in the room, and at 9:35 I was addressing about 200 members of the Indian Medical Association. As far as I could judge, this was normal. Indeed, everything seemed to go smoothly and in its own sweet way. I was annoyed at myself for having not waited to be picked up and taken there. We would only have been 25 minutes late and therefore in good time!

On December 27, Murray Clark and I set off to see the Kali Temple, partly for its own sake, but also to look for Mother Theresa's Mission for the Destitute and Dying, which is housed in an old temple owned by the Kali Temple. Possibly 200 people were lying on couches, a party of religious sisters were changing dry dressings and food was being prepared in a large cauldron. We met a West German student doing social work instead of the requisite military service. He told me that the turnover of patients was pretty fast because 50 per cent of the people on the beds die within a couple of days of admission. There was evidence of love and an abundance of hot food—fortified soup—but no medical or real cure-directed treatment. Anyone can just turn up to help in the mission and, if they ask to help, some sort of job will be found. There is, of course, no pay.

As I think back to this 1974 visit, I am reminded of comments made in Edmonton 15 years or so later by an Alberta nurse who had visited the Kali Temple refuge. She was quite critical of the fact that there was no attempt to give even such simple therapy as intravenous fluid to those too weak to eat. She had a point. Mother Theresa, for years, showed tenderness and care, but could she not have harnessed volunteer medical help, along the lines of Médecins Sans Frontières? It is food for thought. Truly those we saw, that day in 1974, were in a sorry and pitiful state but I remember no feelings of responsibility for their helplessness—just pathos.

By contrast the next morning, my last in Calcutta, I went across Calcutta in a chauffeur-driven car to the new Bellevue Clinic, a private hospital, to see a 49-year-old woman with a kidney problem. I certainly agreed with the diagnosis and that the management was correct. As I passed out of the room, the patient's nephew pressed an envelope into my hand. Later I found out that my consultation had been rewarded by 500 rupees, prepared in advance—what a place! After lunch, I flew to Madras, where I was met by Dr. K.V. Johny, the nephrologist at Vellore.

MADRAS AND VELLORE

That night at the Arun Hotel in Madras, a reception was hosted by the local army commander, a navy commander and their wives. During dinner, I was asked if I would join two of the wives in judging the beauty contest. How could I refuse? All five women were quite lovely. I picked numbers one, two and five, then there was a reshuffle and the final order was two, one and three. Then, under the flood lights and the occasional

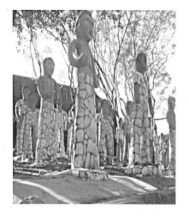

On a side-trip to Chandrigarh in Punjab, I visited this famous garbage dump. The caretaker has made hundreds of figures and animals from broken glass bangles, broken crockery, broken earthenware fuse boxes, telegraph pole spreaders, metal soft drink bottle tops, broken crockery mugs, empty tar barrels and excess building materials of all sorts. This garden of primitive art is truly aesthetically satisfying. I am sure that when the moon is full and the soft smell of jasmine hangs in the air, all these figures come to life and move, stiffly at first, but then ever more loosely as the concrete softens, to finally cavort around in reels, quadrilles and fandangos. Hours later, a cock must crow and the concrete starts to harden again and all returns to normal just before dawn.

flash, I was charmingly invited to crown the queen. Should I give her a kiss on the cheek? She was certainly very lovely. My last minute decision was No. It soon became clear that was correct!

The next morning we drove to Vellore and I spent most of the day—until 4.30 p.m.—touring the Christian Medical College, seeing the dialysis unit and giving a talk to the staff. My talk seemed to be well received, although it was hard to gauge; I think the audience of 50 had varied medical backgrounds. Anticipating this, I had put together a potpourri of straight clinical internal medicine, sprinkled with dialysis and transplantation, and finished with our research.

January and September 1981

My first stop in January 1981 was to visit Dr. Hargovind Laxmishankar Trivedi at his new position in Ahmedabad, the sixth largest city in India. Trivedi was a nephrologist who had practiced for ten years in North America, including two years of nephrology/transplant training at The Cleveland Clinic, and then eight years of nephrology practice in Canada, which is where I had come to know him. After becoming settled in a comfortable position in Hamilton, Ontario, he journeyed to Ahmedabad, his old school, for a sabbatical leave. There he became convinced that his future lay back in India, so he returned. They, of course, were delighted to have him and he found himself the only kidney specialist for 49 million people. I visit him whenever I get to India.

I returned to India in September 1981, primarily to give a two-day workshop on transplantation in Bombay with Dr. Phil Belitsky, a urologist and transplant surgeon from Dalhousie University, at the meeting of the Indian Urology Association in Bombay. But first, I took a quick trip to Ahmedabad to see Trivedi. Of course, it was more than a social call.

On my first day, I was up at five to sort the slides in preparation for a talk on the HLA system, and was then whisked off to the B.J. Medical College and Civil Hospital (a public institution), to see four renal patients: two with acute renal failure, one with a glucose-6phosphate G deficiency, and the other a woman with partial cortical necrosis of kidneys from post-partum sepsis and shock. I then saw two girls with nephrotic syndrome, one membranous, the other with minimal lesion nephrotic syndrome. We discussed these people's problems at length.

All the nephrology trainees read the *New England Journal Medicine* and were up-to-date clinically, but there were other limitations. There was no proper charting of patient data, no blood gas measurements, no follow-up clinic after discharge, and no advanced stains for their kidney biopsies. In addition, microscope sections were cut too thick for good definition. On the plus side, there were many unusual clinical cases of kidney disease of great interest on the public wards.

The public wards were in a shameful state. Mattresses were ragged with holes, bedpans were chipped and gruesome smells from the morgue wafted through one end of the hospital. Families of villagers crouched all over the place throughout day and night, providing much of the ward care and all the meals. Birds flitted around everywhere in the long wards. I had to assume that all this was acceptable, even normal, though I could not help thinking about the reaction of a head nurse, ward sister or matron of a teaching hospital in the Western hemisphere!

The physicians had chloroquine (Aralen—an anti-malaria drug), benzodiazepines (Diazepam), penicillin, sulpha drugs and lots of prednisone. Prednisone seems always to be plentiful.

I would have liked to have stayed longer but I had my talk on the HLA system, which went well, although everyone seemed surprised when I stopped on time.

After lunch, I accompanied Trivedi on a one-hour drive to Gandinager— the seat of the Gujarat government—to see the Gujarat minister of health. Trivedi was heavily involved in state politics in an effort to get a public kidney hospital started. The minister at Gandinager held court seated at a large desk with chairs arranged around it in two semicircles. Anyone can get to see him without an appointment. He makes decisions and writes his answer across the memoranda or briefs and hands them back. He is a one man *panchayat*, a bit like the district officer meting out justice in the days of the Raj, except that instead of sitting under a spreading banyan tree he is ensconced in a cathedral of bureaucracy.

Trivedi gave an account of our joint plans for a University of Alberta and Ahmedabad connection in renal research, and I supplemented his account. It was sympathetically received and he asked all the right questions. Eventually, the government of Gujarat helped Trivedi with his ambitious plans. Together, a few years later, we sent equipment to help established a transplant immunology laboratory and the nine-month loan of one of our senior Edmonton transplant technicians, Sue Saidman (now Sue Saidman, PhD). It seemed right to share our expertise.

Back in Bombay for the two-day medical-surgical workshop on kidney transplantation, I was assaulted by the discomfort and squalor of the slums, which must be even worse in the monsoon season. There were no drains, no sidewalks, no sewage, no waterproof roofing. When about 12 cm (five inches) of rains falls in 48 hours, the whole slum is ankle deep in greenish-brown liquid, which is malodorous to boot. Meanwhile, we stayed at the magnificent Taj Mahal Hotel. Again, there was that bewildering contrast of rich and poor. One hopes never to take it for granted.

The first day of the workshop focused on transplantation immunology and the HLA system, from 9:00 a.m. to 6.30 p.m., after which I consulted on a patient. The second day focused on surgical issues and lasted until 3:00 p.m. Burroughs Wellcome (who made the immunosuppressant azathioprine [Imuran]) were co-sponsors of the whole affair. We were successful in pulling together doctors in the various kidney transplant groups across India to discuss their experiences. Altogether it was deemed a great success.

January 4–12, 2000

It is not often that a person realizes his or her long-cherished dream, but one who has had this satisfaction is my friend, Trivedi. In 1977, when Trivedi returned to Ahmedabad after giving up a prosperous practice of nephrology in Canada, he conceived the idea of an autonomous kidney and transplant centre within the confines of the B.J. Medical College and Civic Hospital. In 1985, it was formed, although it did not truly become a reality until 1992 or so. Now the Institute for Kidney Disease and Research Centre (IKDRC) is a going concern and a magnificent tribute to Trivedi's integrity, determination, political skills and ability to raise the millions of rupees necessary to build an initial 250-bed research hospital, which later expanded to 400 beds.

Perhaps even more remarkable than the existence of this institute is the fact that it has contributed remarkable things to the world of research and the acquisition of new knowledge. One simply does not expect flashes of new discoveries in applied science in India—primarily because of the expense of ancillary laboratory and diagnostic facilities and the financial support of the experts to run them. However, the work at the institute is very good, and carried out with integrity and great clinical skill.

They achieved a breakthrough with live related kidney transplantations by using bone marrow-derived primitive cells (now called adult-derived stem cells). These cells are released into the circulation of prospective kidney donors in response to an injected stimulus, and then harvested from removed blood using a procedure called plasmapheresis. Here, the white cellular elements are removed, the plasma and red blood cells returned and the white cells are injected into the prospective recipients. This procedure of white blood cell removal from prospective kidney donors is performed several times each week for about a month before transplantation. This induces what they think (and I agree) is donor-specific immunological tolerance to the donor kidney. This state of immunologic tolerance is achieved by what is known as micro-chimerism—the co-existence of two immune systems (donor and recipient) at the same time in the post-transplant recipient. These patients do not need as many immunosuppressive drugs post-operatively, have fewer post-transplant infections and are a lot less likely to reject the organ.

Would this research have passed a Canadian Research Ethics Board (REB)? Probably not. But then in Canada, the director of the research program is not the chair of the REB. Their success, however, in terms of the percentage of surviving grafts, is striking. After more than 100 patients over an 18-month period, the protocol seems to be really working and I am most impressed and pleased for them. They submitted a paper to the *New England Journal of Medicine*, but it was not accepted. However, Trivedi was invited to give an address on their work at the 19th meeting of the International Transplant Society in Miami in August 2002.[75]

These improved outcomes will lead to an increase in the frequency of live-related-donor transplants in the rest of the world, especially in the less industrialized world, where cadaveric donor programs are too expensive and have less appeal, and where kidney commerce has flourished—even when illegal.

By 2000, my knowledge of nephrology and transplantation immunology was rusty, to say the least. So what was I doing at the IKDRC transplantation meeting? Well, unlike nephrology and other specialties, one's knowledge of medical ethics does not deteriorate as readily with age, and such discussions are relevant to any medical congress. It was my good fortune to be invited to this congress to talk about the ethics of transplantation, contrasting the West's issues with those in the developing world. I also participated in a panel discussion of ethics issues in intensive care units, and when to use cardiopulmonary resuscitation. The issues are much the same in India as in the West, except that the concept of personal autonomy is not as strong, and therefore the concepts of informed consent and advance directives are not as dominant.

The conference was enjoyable to me for another reason. One of the speakers was Dr. Susan Saidman, then head of Transplant Immunology at Massachusetts General Hospital, but previously one of the technicians in our lab in Edmonton. She is well known in Ahmedabad because of her work there 17 years previously when she established a transplant immunology lab as part of a good will gesture from the University of Alberta.

Shortly after the Congress ended, I was taken to the airport to begin the long trek back to Ottawa. I thought it was the end of my Indian academic trips—my veritable swan song—but it was not quite.

What is the state of medical ethics in India?

My exposure to medical ethics in India has been through relationships with physicians and, to a lesser extent, with some of their medical problems. My dealings with sick people has been very limited, as has my participation in bedside discussions where the person's individual dilemmas are discussed. Nor do I speak Hindustani or any of the many other languages of India. It is therefore very likely that I have had insufficient exposure to Indian medicine to make valid comments on its ethics. Nonetheless, here are my views formed during my eight visits between 1974 and 2000.

Medical ethics in academic circles in India bears similarities to the Western professional ethics I experienced as a medical student some 50 years ago. There was an assumption then that one would do the right thing for patients, modelled on the precepts of one's teachers, but actual debate on ethical issues seldom occurred, and there was very little discussion about what an individual patient thought in a given dilemma. This has now completely changed in North America and Europe, where ethics issues are discussed all the time, using the language of ethics (every physician in the West understands this new language, though admittedly few are entirely comfortable using it). This is not yet the case in India, although I am sure it is heading in the same directions.

Whose health ethics? Based on what premises?

Physicians in India have varied backgrounds: Hindu, Muslim, Christian and Western science or secular. This is the root of the East/West paradox. Clearly, when interacting with physicians in such fields as hemodialysis and kidney transplantation, Indian physicians are familiar with Western training and experience, including exposure to Western bioethics. Most physicians in India speak excellent English and Indian medical literature is comparable to that of the West. But the large majority are also Hindu, and this endows them with a commitment to tolerance and ethical reflection (as well, regrettably, to passive acceptance of the Hindu caste system). My conclusion is that this gives them an ethical system that they would probably *express* in Western syntax—if they verbalized it at all— but think about in term of Eastern spirituality.

Table 9.1 summarizes the differences I perceive between medical ethics in the East and those in the West.

However, there is an upsurge of interest in bioethics in the economically developing world, which will lead, in my view, to significant changes in how we see our Western ethics systems. It may well come from a dialectic between the two systems, one based on ethical principle, personal autonomy and law, the other on spirituality and relationships with others and with nature, synthesized into a global ethic that incorporates the best of both systems.

A step in this evolution is the work done in relational ethics, initiated and published by Prof. Vangie Bergum[76] at the University of Alberta, in which research I was privileged to play a part. I subscribe to the view that health ethics in the West has become overly confrontational and legalistic and to that extent, I agree wholeheartedly with the Eastern perspective.

On the other hand, health ethics in the East—to the extent that one can talk about a single system at all—may need to strengthen its commitment to the concept of primacy of the individual person, restraint on

Table 9.1 Some philosophical differences between Eastern and Western bioethics.

Typical Western view	The Eastern view
1. Focus is on the individual in ethics and law	1. Focus is on community, family and extended family
2. Religious dogma no longer the dominant ethic	2. More awareness of nature, spirituality and the I environment—but no religious dogma
3. Dilemmas are decided on precedent and context	3. Relationships preferred to rights
4. Minority opinion is respected because of commitment to human rights	4. Ethics is "love for life"
5. Autonomy is king in matters of consent	5. Ethics is dialogue
6. Respect the Golden Rule	6. Respect the Golden Rule
	7. View Western bioethics as confrontational

paternalism (whether exercised by senior family members, professionals, community leaders or government), gender equality and natural human rights based on the equality of each person's moral worth.

The ultimate ethical dilemma in health care: resource allocation

Resource allocation in the context of health care seems to depend on:

- the attitudes of a society or culture toward each of its members, especially those who are least advantaged in the lottery of life;
- the overall financial resources (wealth) of the society as a whole; and
- how that wealth is controlled, or shared, by private interests or corrupt regimes, on the one hand, and a sense of the common good as implemented by non-corrupt regimes, on the other.

Compare, if you will, contemporary health delivery in resource-rich areas of the developing world. For example, the factor that characterizes Singapore is a commitment by a non-corrupt government to extending health entitlement to everyone in the society; whereas in Brunei, an equally rich country, personal wealth, patronage, and powerful connections are the main determinants of entitlement and the less advantaged members of society miss out.

It is arguably not merely happenstance that Singapore is democratic and does not have a dominant political ethic based in a religious hierarchy, whereas Brunei is a hegemony with a religious system that is intricately meshed with the power of the state.

Some resource-poor countries in the developing world provide public health measures, such as immunization programs and safe drinking water. But none of them can afford to extend health entitlement to all (one only has to think of sub-Saharan Africa). Thus, the main factors in providing health care to those in most need are increasing overall national wealth (e.g., lowering trade barriers, facilitating local manufacturing), and monitoring the nature and integrity of government. (Another dreadful aspect is that so many of these poor countries spend disproportionate amounts of national wealth on armaments made in the West.)

India is a democratic country—in fact the world's most populous democracy—with a relatively non-corrupt government, but it does not have resources to extend entitlement to health care to all its citizens. But relative to sub-Saharan Africa and its totally overwhelming HIV/AIDS epidemic, India has many resources, and thus holds the middle ground in the rich-poor spectrum. Among its approximately 1 billion citizens, only about 50 million people (5%) can afford some sort of health care beyond that offered through publicly funded hospitals, and only ten million (1%) can afford Western style health care—such as dialysis and kidney transplantation. (Note: Infant mortality stands at 80/1,000, whereas Canada's is only 5.2/1,000; and India's overall density of population per square km is 300, compared with three in Canada.)

Apart from the inequity of the caste system and other aspects of Hinduism (80% of Indians are Hindu), it is clear that health for all citizens is quite beyond the reach of India's resources. This is also true for the majority of Muslims on the subcontinent—144 million in Pakistan, and another 108 million in India.

This being the case, another important question arises: If it is clear that a country's resources cannot extend health entitlement to all its citizens, what then is the ethical duty of those who practice contemporary Western medical science in such a country?

This, of course, is Trivedi's dilemma at the Kidney Institute. The conclusion he came to, and it is one to which I subscribe, can be summarized as follows: "I may not be able to be a part of a universal health care system, as I was in Canada, but on returning to my native country, do I go into public health, or become a sewage engineer, or do I continue trying to do what I am specially trained to do—treat persons with kidney failure—in as just and equitable a manner as possible?"

He took the latter route. After he had obtained funding for an autonomous kidney research and treatment centre (which in 2001 grew from 250 to 400 beds) within the government-supported Civil Hospital, he keeps things operational by using the following financial strategy: 20 per cent of the beds are for wealthy patients who pay Western rates for Western-type care. The profit from this, together with government and other private and corporate funding sources, is sufficient to offer the remaining 80 per cent of beds to indigent patients, free of charge. Of course, 400 beds for dialysis and renal transplantation is a mere drop in a bucket in relation to renal failure needs of the 49 million people the centre serves, but what more can one do? Trivedi does what he can and that is what he perceives as his ethical duty.

In many ways his situation mirrors that faced by the late Mother Theresa at her Mission for the Destitute and Dying. The one can be criticized for doing too much, the other too little. The dilemmas of ethics were ever like this. Each must face this dilemma in his or her own way; there is no right answer. At best, one can live in accordance with Albert Schweitzer's concept of reverence for life.

III. A career in ethics

In every system of morality…I have always remarked that the author proceeds for some time in the ordinary way of reasoning,…or makes observations concerning human affairs when all of a sudden I am surprised to find that, instead of the usual copulation of propositions "is" and "is not," I meet with no proposition that is not connected with an "ought" or "ought not." This change is imperceptible, but it is however of the last [ultimate] consequence. For as this "ought" or "ought not" expresses some new relation or affirmation it is necessary that it should be explained and, at this same time, that a reason should be given for what seems altogether inconceivable: how this new relation can be a deduction from others which are entirely different from it.

David Hume (1711–1776)
Treatise on Human Nature, III, I, I

10

Sabbatical in ethics, 1985–1986: Getting from "is" to "ought"

WITH THE GROWTH IN GENERAL medical knowledge in the second half of the 20th century and my experiences in nephrology, which touched on one small part of that growth, came an increasing awareness of health ethics, both in professional health care practice and clinical research. Ultimately, this led to a significant change in my career direction from medical practice into health ethics (also called bioethics or medical ethics).

My gradual awakening to the ethical hazards of end-stage kidney disease in both dialysis and organ transplantation was accompanied by a growing dissatisfaction with the intensity and efficacy of our research. In saying "our," I am speaking for the efforts of the applied section of the transplant group at the University of Alberta. We had become increasingly separate from the basic science section and it was clear that we were no longer in symbiosis, which had been the original intention. This was a considerable disappointment to me, as I had genuinely believed that an alliance between a basic and a clinical science researcher (Erwin Diener and myself) could result in something spectacular in the new field of transplant immunology. Research, however, evolves in unpredictable ways, with the basic scientist wanting to get more basic, and the applied clinical scientist needing to remain clinically relevant. I also found that as I grew older—particularly after the age of 55—my administrative responsibilities began to dilute my dedication to research, especially that dedication needed to keep up to date with one's reading of new scientific findings in the literature. Thus, I felt that we had lost the cutting edge, scientifically.

But there were also some positive drivers behind the impetus to change my career, stemming from my increasing conviction that some physicians may be involved in practices that do not always give patients the opportunities for health restoration that they deserve. This seemed to be a matter for great ethical concern. In my practice of nephrology, the following four examples come to mind.

1. *Ought not all nephrologists to feel remorse that for a decade and a half—almost to the end of the 1970s—people reaching the end stage of kidney failure from longstanding diabetes were not offered the benefit of dialysis or transplantation? Then it was shown that they could be effectively maintained by dialysis and even do well after cadaver kidney transplantation.*

   The short answer is yes, but the standard answer and rationale at that time was that: (a) the placing of vascular access devices in their arms—where diabetes had already caused peripheral arterial disease—would lead to gangrene of fingers and precipitate amputations, and (b) placing these people on anticoagulants during dialysis—a necessary step—could worsen diabetic retinopathy and lead to retinal hemorrhage and blindness. These factors led to a policy whereby persons with diabetic end-stage renal failure were simply not referred to nephrologists for an opinion on their suitability for dialysis. When a small minority of dialysis physicians insisted that these people be fully treated, it was soon shown that this rationale was not evidence-based and that such people ought to, and indeed did, do well. A decade later, the largest single group of newcomers to dialysis were diabetic kidney patients.

2. *Ought not nephrologists in charge of kidney dialysis units to ensure that all dialysis patients are referred for transplantation assessment as soon as they become stable on dialysis? And should they not be indifferent to the possible loss of income as their patients move out of dialysis?*

   The short answer is yes, all patients should be immediately referred. The failure to refer may be more prevalent in units that are controlled by dialysis manufacturing firms, where physician-directors may receive salaries from these firms.

3. *Since the value of cadaveric organ transplantation has been so palpably demonstrated, ought not nephrologists and other*

physicians, including all family physicians, to become advocates for organ and tissue donation and spend more time discussing the risks and benefits with patients? Is it not unethical if they fail to advocate for this vital need, claiming, perhaps, that it is not part of the professional obligation of every physician?

Again, the short answer is yes. However, polls show that even though almost all people (more than 80 per cent) favour the use of organs for transplantation after death, relatively few (about 33 per cent) have actually signed donor cards or registered their support through advance directives. Family physicians and other specialists who look after patients who are planning their future health decision-making, or who are suffering from potentially fatal conditions, could help greatly to overcome this natural inertia, yet they do not do so.

4. *Who is responsible for deciding which person on a transplant waiting list ought to receive a cadaveric kidney when one is available? Where does that authority come from? By what principles ought that allocation to be made?*

There is no short answer to these questions; they require careful thought and policy decision-making.

As my career progressed, I felt an increasing desire to study the ethics processes by which decisions are made in practice. How should we to go about making decisions in these and similar situations? In line with David Hume's thought, which opened this chapter, I wanted to study the ways by which the "is," that is, the factual realities of everyday clinical affairs, could become the "ought," the underlying values that should guide decisions. As Hume pointed out, the transition from "is" to "ought" is profound, yet everyone is obliged to make such transitions every day.

I was also struck by the fact that patients' decision-making—making good or bad choices for dialysis—was an increasingly significant concern. Many individuals—particularly those over 70 years of age—made what seemed to be bad choices for themselves when presented with the unrestricted dialysis options available to them. The correlative issue for nephrologists and others was how to recognize those who would do well on dialysis and guide them in that direction. They also had to learn how to recognize those who would probably not do well, and not paint an overly optimistic picture of the benefits of that would ensue. It was too easy, I thought, to advocate for *simple longevity*, when what patients really want is *optimal quality of life*. The dilemma is further compounded with ethical risk when the physician's earnings are promoted by the dialysis process.

Quality of Life Committee

With these thoughts in mind, I invited some colleagues to join me in forming a Quality of Life Committee in 1984. This group consisted of a vice-director of nursing, a professor of nursing, two members of the clergy, a dialysis nurse, a philosopher trained in bioethics, and a health law professor, who later became a justice of the Court of Queen's Bench. We met on the ward where we had the patient's records and, occasionally, we met with patients. The committee discussed with them the details of their life on dialysis and the difficult circumstances that the treatment regimen presented to them, including:

- the fluid intake restrictions;
- the maintenance of the arterio-venous silastic-tube loops inserted in arm vessels, which are broken open thrice-weekly to connect to the hemodialysis machine;
- the discomforts of fluid overload from simply drinking too much fluid of any sort for those with borderline congestive heart failure;
- the tedium of travelling for thrice-weekly six-hour dialysis sessions; and
- the more serious complications that led to shunt infections, pneumonias, or heart failure.

Despite these hazards, some did remarkably well for years on end. Others, especially older people, did poorly and had a quality of life that was low and medically complicated. Some were put on peritoneal dialysis, where tubes are placed, on a semi-permanent basis, into the peritoneal cavity of the abdomen and the intra-peritoneal space is used for fluid exchanges on a continuous basis, ridding the body of nitrogen end-products by that route.

Ethical Dilemma

One example of the ethical dilemmas the committee struggled with—an example I purposely chose because it has a good ending—was the case of a 72-year-old gentleman, J.P. (initials have been changed). He experienced many complications on hemodialysis, so was switched, after a year of treatment, to peritoneal dialysis in his second year. Unfortunately, he then suffered recurrent bouts of peritonitis, abdominal pain, lack of appetite, and required repeated courses of antibiotics. He lost 18 kilograms (40 pounds) and was miserable, though uncomplaining.

One day, a 62-year-old patient died from a stroke and the family gave permission for his kidneys to be used. Prior to his death, the donor had some elevation of blood pressure, evidence of diffuse arterial disease and some reduction in overall kidney function. It was decided, on group reflection, that we should not offer this organ to younger patients on the program who were stable on dialysis. However, one of my colleagues, J.P.'s long-term nephrologist, thought J.P. should be asked if he wanted to escape peritoneal dialysis, albeit by accepting a kidney of dubious quality.

J.P. was over the age limit at which patients were considered suitable for transplantation[*] but he was dying a slow death in our hands. The risks were carefully explained. He then disclosed that his wife had had a stroke that affected her speech. He could understand her, but others had great difficulty. He wanted to live as long as possible because she needed him as her interpreter. He promptly accepted the suboptimal organ.

To everyone's delight, not least his own, he did very well. He did not show much rejection activity from his immune system—a phenomenon since recognized more widely with older people—and therefore did not need high doses of immunosuppressive agents. Nor did he develop infections with those strange organisms to which transplant recipients are

---

[*] As previously noted, the upper age for acceptability for transplantation had been rising in rough proportion to the increasing age of dialysis and transplantation program directors.

particularly prone. He regained his appetite and 14 kilograms (30 pounds), and felt well. Indeed, he lived another eight years with a well-functioning kidney.

This experience raised a further question: *Ought* age alone be a determinant of health care entitlement? The short answer in Canada is no. Indeed, a few years later, a group in Norway showed that among patients without chronic disease, those over 70 who received a kidney transplant did well compared with those in the younger age groups.[77] Recently, I reviewed the subject of age-based limitation of health care entitlement for transplantation and found the practice to be unethical.[78]

This question may well become a cultural concern, as increasing numbers of people require expensive technologies to prolong their lives. The debate is heated on both sides. The former director of the Hastings Center for Health Ethics, Daniel Callahan, continues to defend his view that when one can say that the "biography of one's life is now largely written," and can acknowledge that one has "almost run the course of life," health care entitlement should become one of *care* and not *cure*. Others, of course, say that this "reeks of ageism."[79]

These were the sorts of problems that the Quality of Life Committee deliberated. It became clear that since these decisions are not solely medical (they also involve psychosocial and spiritual aspects), physicians need help as they try to work through the transition from is to ought with the patients.

The one person on the nephrology team who has special insight into the psychosocial and spiritual needs of the patients is the dialysis/ nephrology nurse. Physicians simply do not know the dialysis patients in the same way as the nurses who care for them over what can be a five- to 15-year period. In the dialysis unit, the whole nursing-patient group are a family. Over the years, the people on dialysis came to depend on those who look after them during the process and on those in adjacent beds, or who are dialysed with them on the same shift. In this branch of health care, nurses stay involved for long periods of time—usually decades— and are the core of expert caring around which the whole program revolves. They are not always given credit for their expertise, but nephrologists truly know. After all, ethics is relationship! (This is a theme that will be discussed further in the last chapter.)

Small wonder that we developed a special role for nephrology nurses at the University Hospital in Edmonton by finding special funding for a nephrology nurse clinician (NNC) program. These NNCs were the backbone of the whole program, which looked after an increasing number of people with kidney failure—they numbered 500 in 1985 (up from 30 or so in 1970). The number has risen much further since then, despite the financial restrictions that came in the 1990s.

Despite this recognition of the role played by the NNCs and the success of the Quality of Life Committee, I still felt something more was needed to lessen the gap between medicine and ethics. This all came home to me with the following event.

A triggering event

One of the most vexing aspects of kidney transplantation is the shortage of kidneys for transplantation. This brings up a complex conflict among several principles, including *personal autonomy* (the right to do more or less what one wants, provided it hurts no one else); the *duty of society* to preserve those values that contribute to the common good of society; the importance of *protecting the most vulnerable* from exploitation by those with power and influence; and the *ethical obligations of third parties* (i.e., health professionals) not to compromise their commitment to society in their efforts to satisfy the wishes of individual members of that society.

About a year after the Quality of Life Committee was formed, this conflict was embodied in one case that soon led me to resign my position as director of Nephrology and Clinical Immunology and expose myself intensively to medical ethics during a sabbatical.

In 1985, J.C. (initials have been changed), a 43-year-old Canadian businessman, had been on dialysis for three years. During most of this time, he was on a waiting list for cadaver kidney transplantation. His dialysis was moderately free of problems, but he found the dialysis seriously impaired his efficiency and his business was languishing. As his frustration mounted, he decided to try something different. He placed an advertisement in the city newspaper stating that he would give $10,000 to any healthy person who would give him a kidney. The story was picked up by the national media and within a few days he had made contact with about 200 potential donors.

His actions had not gone unnoticed by the local renal transplant program and his dialysis physician got in touch with him to point out that what he had proposed was actually against Canadian law. In essence, he told me this was all very well, but in a free society, he should be able buy a kidney if someone was willing to sell him one. He saw this as another paternalistic denial of basic human rights, but since it was law, he said he was willing to accept it. He decided to re-advertise, saying that he was mistaken in not knowing the law, and that he had no intention of leading anyone who contacted him into a false situation or legal compromise; he asked for someone to donate a kidney out of love!

I said this would not do either: "We would not do a mutilating operation to remove a kidney from someone you did not previously know or who did not know you. Our policy is to use kidneys from living donors only if they are family members or have a strong emotional attachment—what we call genetic or emotional ties."

J.C.'s level of indignation rose another notch. He demanded to know who gave me the right to make the rules by which his life had to be lived? He cited this as yet another example of the arrogance that doctors show towards those who challenge their control of things.

There the matter rested for a while. He then presented a list of six people from across Canada who were prepared to give him a kidney out of love. Each had written a clear expression of intent, stating that they knew what they were doing, that no money would be accepted, and they had no ill health nor, specifically, any mental problems such as depression. There was evidence that a template letter had been sent to each. J.C. now challenged the physicians to tell each of these six potential donors why their wish to give a kidney would not be honoured, and to give those reasons in writing.

The renal transplant team had much discussion over this impasse and a new policy was hammered out. Unrelated living donors would be accepted, even in the absence of genetic or emotional ties, if the potential donor agreed (a) to two physical and psychiatric assessments six months apart; and (b) that if a potential donor had a spouse, a letter of agreement from the spouse would be requested (but not made a binding condition). J.C. said that this policy was an attempt to make things difficult for the potential donors, all of whom lived in other parts of Canada and who would have to pay for the whole process. Nevertheless, he agreed. Several potential donors had an initial assessment.

Five-and-a-half months later, J.C. received a well-matched cadaver kidney and did well post-operatively. Another dialysis patient was overheard to say, "One way to jump the line, huh?"

Ethical Dilemma

When carried out under optimal conditions, the living kidney donor has a very low complication rate and usually lives a normal life. This claim is now based on 40 years of experience. So what is wrong with selling a kidney, when most Western countries allow individuals to sell sperm, ova and blood? What is the justification for not paying donors when everyone else in the field (surgeons, physicians, nurses, social workers, transplant co-ordinators, etc.) is compensated for their time and effort?

I found these dilemmas to be very challenging, and it brought me to a realization that I needed to study, and to think more deeply, about the restriction that ethics and the law imposed, in most Western countries, on commerce in organs and tissues.

A medical ethics sabbatical, 1985–1986

Although the Quality of Life Committee was useful for addressing ethical issues at the bedside, the increasing complexity of these issues led me to believe that deeper education for students and clinicians was also essential and propelled me into a career change at the age of 60.

Medical ethics is not of recent origin. That would be doing great injustice to Hippocrates in ancient Greece, Moses Maimonides (born Cordova, 1135; buried Tiberius, 1204) in the North African Arab culture of the 12th century, or Thomas Perceval in 18th and early 19th century England, whose writings were used as the foundation for the first American Medical Association Code of Ethics in 1847, and so on.

Two long traditions have merged. The first was expressed by the dedication of religious orders and organizations, such as the Knights Templar during the Middle Ages and subsequent nursing orders, to creating hospitals, or hospices, in which to look after "our Lords, the sick." The second grew from increasing medical competency spurred by the Enlightenment (from, say, 1600) as information about diseases and their mechanisms of causation began to accrue. Both traditions claimed ethical centrality for the doctor-patient relationship.

In our third epoch of medical progress (1940–2000), medical ethics radically changed and continues to change. Previously, it was seen as the purview of the medical profession and was much conflated with medical etiquette (quite another subject). In recent decades, the delivery of health care has became more powerful, more capable of doing good and more capable of doing harm. This has led to new dilemmas of ethical conflict in completely unprecedented circumstances. Should one tell dying patients that their outlook is medically hopeless? Is it right to inhibit ovulation so that pregnancy cannot occur with sexual intercourse? Since suicide has ceased to be condemned by our society as a sin and a crime, should assisting another person's suicide always be considered morally and legally wrong? Is it acceptable to use organs from someone who has died to prolong the life in another person, or is it a form of desecration and impiety toward the recently deceased? At the end of life, does not the desire to prolong another's life also entail careful consideration of the quality of life that is being provided?

In earlier chapters, I discussed some of the big-ticket ethical dilemmas I have faced in four decades of practice and the ways in which I tried to address them, or failed to recognize them. I will also devote an entire chapter to research ethics because it is, and continues to be, so replete with its own big-ticket examples of ethical debate.

I will not deal directly with the innumerable small-ticket ethical issues faced almost every day, but they are no less important. In the clinical context, an example of these issues is the respect for patients as shown in:

- how patients are addressed;
- how patients are greeted in office or consultation;
- how to offset the distancing effect of the white coat culture;
- how to maintain a commitment to respect patients when they are asked to meet the physician for the first time wearing a shapeless gown loosely tied at the back;
- how to maintain a commitment for collaborative, participatory, decision-making in physician-patient encounters where time is rationed to the minimum; and
- the issue of personal honesty in disclosure of all relevant facts in seeking "comprehended consent," a wider concept than "informed consent."

These small-ticket ethics issues—and the above examples are merely a tiny sampling of them—are vitally important to a humane health system and would assume a large portion of this text if its purpose was to write a text on ethics for health professionals. Instead, I will focus on the big-ticket—the life or death—ethical conundrums that are of interest to a wider audience, including the legal profession and philosophy students.

AN ANNOTATED BIBLIOGRAPHY OF
MY EARLY READINGS IN ETHICS

Core resources

T.L. Beauchamp, *Philosophical Ethics*[80]

T.L. Beauchamp, J. Childress, *Principles of Biomedical Ethics*[81]

Texts of biomedical ethics

E.D. Pellegrino and D.C. Thomasma, *A Philosophical Basis of Medical Practice: Toward a Philosophy and Ethic of the Healing Professions*[82]

C. Gilligan, *In a Different Voice, Psychological Theory and Women's Development*[83,84]

H. Tristram Engelhardt, *Foundations of Bioethics*[85]

Alasdair MacIntyre, *A Short History of Ethics: A History of Moral Philosophy from the Homeric Age to the Twentieth Century*[86]

Daniel Callahan, *Setting Limits: Medical Goals in an Ageing Society*[87]

A.R. Jonsen, S. Toulmin, *The Abuse of Casuistry: A History of Moral Reasoning*[88]

A.R. Jonsen, M. Seigler, W. Winslade *Clinical Ethics: A Practical Approach to Ethical Decisions in Clinical Medicine*[89]

Peter Singer, *Ethics*[90]

Peter Singer, *Applied Ethics*[91]

Peter Singer, *The Expanding Circle: Ethics and Sociobiology*[92]

Helga Kuhse, Peter Singer, *Should the Baby Live? The Problem of Handicapped Infants*[93]

John Finnis, *Natural Law and Natural Rights*[94]

Bernard Williams, *Ethics and the Limits of Philosophy*[95]

Warren T. Reich, *Encyclopaedia of Bioethics*[96]

John Rawls, *A Theory of Justice*[97]

D.J. Roy, J.R. Williams, B.M. Dickens, *Bioethics in Canada*[98]

In pursuit of knowledge

Many would consider that, in 1985, I was almost completely unprepared for leadership in medical ethics at a medical school. I shared that view and it caused me much introspection at the time. What would be the required preparation for that sort of venture? Was I not being pretentious to embark on such a course? Obviously, in order to undertake such a task, one needs to know about health care and the dilemmas faced at the bedside. That part I had experienced. However, I had never studied philosophy per se, so I set about changing that by reading. Though by no means exhaustive, the list on page 173 indicates lists some of the texts that guided me.

I also delved into resources such as the *Hastings Center Reports*, the *Journal of Medical Ethics*, the *Journal of Clinical Ethics*, *The Cambridge Quarterly Journal*, and ethics articles in the *New England Journal of Medicine* and *JAMA*.

While reading extensively about ethics I wondered whether this would justify my claim to have sufficient insight into ethical decision-making to presume to teach others about it. After all, ethics is a subject in which *everyone* is a practitioner. We all make ethical decisions every day. It is part of being a normal person living in a society. Does studying these practical aspects of ethics lead to ethical probity and practical wisdom? I hope so, although I still do not know for sure. Reading extensively in ethics, however, may:

- impart the language skills to enable the cogent expression of one's views on a subject, using the situations that one has dealt with in the past;
- enable one to lead discussions and exchange views on the ethical aspects of a given dilemma;
- make one aware of which views are based on intuition, not reasoning, and the origin of those intuitions in religious, historical or ideological traditions;
- enable one to develop frameworks for ethical decision-making and conflict resolution that are not narrowly based on religious, historical or ideological traditions but are, rather, based on a system of secular ethics, which, it is hoped, could be shared by all people in a society;
- lead one to acknowledge that decisions about right and wrong conduct should be based, as much as possible, on reasoned principles from which we derive rules;
- lead one also to acknowledge that there is an emotional side—not based on reason—in which emotion, feelings, intuitions and gut reactions all play a legitimate part; and
- make one think about the *interplay* of rules (based on principles) and moral intuitions (based on emotions and conscience) in a dynamic dialectic—an interplay that always takes place within the context of actual *human relationships, circumstances* and *past experiences*. In fact, it is these relationships between people that define what ethics is all about.

Ethics is concerned with making morally correct decisions and taking morally correct actions. It is the process by which we judge actions as right or wrong in relation to a shared set of norms and principles of behaviour embraced by our society as a whole. The foundation of ethics, or "Reverence for Life" is, I believe, that:

1. all humans are moral equals, therefore
2. each should be respected and treated with dignity, so as to
3. promote good human relationships and personal flourishing.

This is not difficult to state, but it is very difficult to apply in specific situations where there is need for conflict resolution concerning principles of conduct. This often requires special knowledge of areas of human conduct, and it is really only this element of professional knowledge of special situations that justifies making a distinction between general ethics, political ethics, business ethics, nursing ethics, community ethics, research ethics, medical ethics and health ethics.

In an effort to augment what I had gleaned from my reading, and to learn as much as possible in as short a period as possible, I decided to spend time with experts at three locations, and to take two bioethics courses at Kennedy Institute of Ethics at Georgetown, Maryland. Thus, in 1985–1986, I spent six weeks with David Roy, PhD, at the Ethics Centre affiliated with the Clinical Research Centre at l'Hôtel Dieu de Montreal; six weeks at the Medical Center in San Francisco, sitting at the feet of Albert Jonsen, PhD, a world-renown ethicist; and four months as a visiting scholar at the Hastings Center, then located at Hastings-on-Hudson, north of New York City. This exposure to different ethicists proved to be increasingly valuable.

In addition to those mentioned above were discussions with my heroes in health ethics: in Canada—John Williams, Bartha Knoppers, Benjamin Freedman, Margaret Somerville, Ted Keyserklingk, Bernard Dickens; in the U.S.—Al Jonsen, Daniel Callahan, Al Caplan, Eva Wolff, Ronald Beyer, Strahan Donnelley, Robert Veatch, Ruth Macklin, Norman Daniels, Dr. Arnold Relman; and that role model for all physicians in medical ethics, Dr. Edmundo Pellegrino.

I have never regretted this decision to redirect my career, except perhaps that I should have made it five years earlier. But in saying that, I am forgetting other aspects of life: two daughters at Atlantic College in Wales, a son in private school on Vancouver Island (until better thinking prevailed and he opted to return to public high school in Edmonton), a third daughter just setting out on a university career, and the house not paid for. Even a geographic full-time medical academic has to consider his or her dependence on clinical earnings. Then there was the fact that such a move would have meant giving up contact with those who shared clinical and research responsibilities with me.

As it turned out, the Medical Research Council agreed to continue my Career Investigatorship for another five years after I switched into medical ethics, an act for which I will always be grateful. In addition, Dr. Douglas Wilson, then dean of medicine at the University of Alberta, graciously supported my request for a sabbatical and my application for a subsistence grant at the three chosen sites and for the Georgetown courses. I could not have been treated more handsomely by all concerned. And then, as always, there was my wife Margaret, who entered enthusiastically into all these plans and came with me for the six weeks in San Francisco.

Teaching ethics to medical students

While in Montreal, San Francisco and New York, I spent time figuring out how to integrate medical ethics into the curriculum of the Faculty of Medicine at the University of Alberta. In this I was in close touch with Glenn Griener, PhD, in our Department of Philosophy. Each evening, I sent my ideas over telnet computer lines into the University of Alberta mainframe for Dalyce Wright, my former secretary at the laboratory and in nephrology who was now also adapting to the world of bioethics, to collate. In fact, she complained I gave her more work while I was on sabbatical than when I was in the office every day. In this way, we prepared to launch our new medical ethics curriculum in September 1986.

I wanted to integrate ethics teaching into each section of the medical curriculum. The underlying idea was to make the ethics curriculum problem-based (or casuistical, for the more philosophically-minded). I did not want the Curriculum Committee to give me a specific number of hours for a separate course in ethics. Instead, I wanted to get each organ system's clinical teaching director (cardiologists, obstetricians, infectious diseases, nephrologists, and the like) to give up some of their allotted teaching time to ethics. Integration would also ensure that health ethics were presented in a clinically-relevant setting or context, avoiding lectures on ethics theory or principle. These, of course, would then be introduced in an inductive process—as distinct from deductive.

The physician director of education for each section agreed to provide space and to present selected dilemmas derived from clinical experiences in their sub-speciality. My colleagues (Griener, Donna Smith, Janet Storch, Fr. Tom Dailey, Justice Ellen Picard, Vangie Bergum and others) and I made up an ethics panel to discuss the main points of each situation. Every panel was led by a physician who knew the patient.

During the summer of 1986, after returning from my sabbatical, I prepared the first edition of the *Teaching Manual in Medical Ethics and Jurisprudence* with assistance from Griener. By September we had all 200 pages ready. The venture was launched initially under the name of the Joint-Faculties Bioethics Project. It was a joint venture because of the heavy involvement of nursing and the collaboration of Dean Janetta MacPhail. It was called a project because we did not want to use any of the words that carry administrative messages in the university such as centre, program, or department. That would all come later.

We also obtained permission from the Curriculum Committee to conduct an examination in ethics. It was allotted five per cent of the yearly marks, and a pass mark was made compulsory. This last step was strongly urged by the students we consulted. They said, "If you don't, it will be seen as Mickey Mouse, and most of the guys will not come to the class, or get interested in it!" (By this time, the term "guys" included both male and female medical students.) I knew they were right.

The exam consisted of an ethical dilemma—similar to some of those presented in this book—which was circulated to all students a week beforehand. They could discuss it among themselves and read any text or article in an effort to get their ideas straight. Then, on the fateful day, they had 40 minutes to write essay answers to three or four questions based on the pre-circulated ethical dilemma. The instructors then assessed these essays and commented on them, after which they were returned to the students. It was a time-consuming but worthwhile process.

We carefully chose big-ticket issues for the medical students. The following would be a suitable dilemma for the exam:

Judge orders girl to have heart swap
M. is 15 years old and will die within a few days if not given a heart transplant. Family, physicians, chaplain and friends all failed to convince her. She is reported to have said,

> "The first I knew about having a transplant was on
> Wednesday. I know what it means: check-ups, tablets for the

rest of your life. I feel depressed about that. I am only 15 and I don't want to take tablets for the rest of my life. It all happened so quickly. If I don't have the operation I will die, I know that.

"But I really don't want a transplant—I am not happy with it. I don't want to die. It's hard to take in. If I had children and they were old enough—say my age—I would go with whatever is best and what they want. Death is final, I know I cannot change my mind. I don't want to die but would rather die than have the transplant and have someone else's heart. I would rather die with 15 years of my own heart. I would feel different with someone else's heart."

Daily Telegraph, London
Friday, July 16, 1999

Was the judge right in ordering the transplant operation against her wishes? What would happen if she refused to take immunosuppressive medication after recovery? Would it be right to force her to take medications?

We also dealt with small-ticket dilemmas. For instance, we asked how a family physician should respond in the following situation:

A physician is treating a young man who is gay, but sees no reason to tell the girl he is about to marry about his sexual preference. The young woman, soon to become his wife, is also that physician's patient.

How should the physician handle this problem? When could the young man's right to confidentiality be overridden by his fiancée's rights to be told the truth, if ever? How would you handle this situation?

Such questions exercise the mind, provoke discussion, make one want to know more about the precise circumstances. These are just the sort of questions that medical students should think about from the viewpoints of principles, intuitions and gut feelings and relationships. Then they should derive their course of action, justify it, and state how they would continue to be involved in and monitor the situation. On the whole, the exams were very well done and everyone passed, year after year.

The activities of the Joint-Faculties Bioethics Project were exciting for me. Much of the time was spent teaching students in small groups on specific issues, or in tackling large classes with a teaching team. As far as possible, I used actual clinical cases as the basis for discussions, selecting them from various sources (including my own experiences) to get to the underlying ethical issues and principles as applied to the clinical context. It seemed to work. The new program increased the medical students' exposure to ethics from six hours jurisprudence before 1985 to more than 40 hours of ethics and jurisprudence during the four-year course.

Such growth could not have taken place without the strong support of the dean of medicine, Douglas Wilson, and subsequently David Lorne Tyrrell; Dr. Neil MacDonald from oncology and Drs. Paul Byrne and David Schiff from pediatrics; the two deans of nursing, Janetta MacPhail and Marilyn Wood, as well as professors of nursing, including Janet Storch, Vangie Bergum, Wendy Austin; Donna Smith, Janet Ross Kerr, Tricia Marck, and Sandy MacPhail; Father Tom Dailey of St. Joseph's College Bioethics Centre; Profs. Cameron McKenzie and Glenn Griener from the Department of Philosophy; Marion Briggs from rehabilitation; Profs. Gerald Robertson, Margaret Shone and Tim Caulfield from the Health Law Centre; Richard Fraser, QC, who was in law practice; Noella Inions, a former nurse who took law and went into health administration; Dr. Tom Noseworthy from Public Health Science, and many others. Success depended on these collaborations, which were always given unstintingly.

These people also served as members of the Steering Committee of the Joint-Faculties Bioethics Project, meeting three or so times a year to discuss the various programs that had been started. Given their involvement in various aspects of teaching, they were not mere advisors; in fact they steered the program throughout the year. Without their support, the new program in bioethics at the University of Alberta would not have succeeded.

Clinical activity after nephrology

When I embarked on this career change, I gave up all my clinical and research activities, relinquishing my position as director of the Division of Nephrology and Clinical Immunology and handing over the direction of the Transplant Immunology Laboratory and its special unit in histocompatibility (tissue typing for transplantation). With my successor, Dr. Phil Halloran, in place, I decided that I should drop out of the immunology/transplantation field. The dialysis program continued to be led by Dr. Raymond Ulan throughout this period of transition, and for another decade or so.

Despite these capable successors, I still had misgivings about relinquishing all my clinical activities, which had been such a dominant part of my life for four decades. Late in 1986, I mentioned this over lunch to my long-time internist friend, Dr. Buzz Edwards, who promptly said, "Join us!" By this he meant join the team of internists who are responsible for the two wards of internal medicine patients (i.e., those internists who did not have a sub-speciality interest rooted in a specific organ system— pulmonologists, gastroenterologists, cardiologists and the like). This seemed a good idea, but did I know enough? He assured me that I did, and that the resident coverage on general internal medicine was very strong. What they needed, he seemed to think, was the "wisdom of the ageing" (I think he meant wisdom of the ages—which is different!).

I decided to try it out, and found that I liked it a lot and it gave me a new clinical experience. My work began during admissions rounds at 7:30 every morning, where the residents who had been on duty during the previous 24 hours brought everyone up to date. I learned a lot at those rounds, and Edwards himself displayed his encyclopaedic knowledge of internal medicine to the advantage of all. I happily shared physician responsibility for the service with Edwards, Peter Hamilton, Bruce Fisher, Dawna Gilchrist, and Leroy (Lee) Anholt. Dr. Garner King, physician-in-chief, attended admission rounds quite often and I came to admire him very much—he was a true leader and a great man. (I was much saddened when he died a few years later of the very condition he had done much to clarify through his research: adult respiratory distress syndrome.)

Edwards was right. There was a need for a physician with some breadth of experience, and it gave me an opportunity to bring medical ethics teaching into the residency training program; I was happy about that. I felt confident of my role, *except* on those rare occasions when the resident was inexperienced. Then I felt exposed and feared somewhat for patient welfare. It was because of this that I felt obliged to give up this clinical responsibility after four years.

Growth of the program

Meanwhile, the health ethics program—and my responsibilities—was continuing to expand.

In addition to teaching, the bioethics group introduced special rounds in clinical ethics at the amphitheatre of the University Hospital on a monthly basis. Situations were presented to nurses, physicians (faculty, attending physicians and residents), and other health professionals and administrators. Some of the topics covered included:

- Should cardiopulmonary resuscitation be withheld sometimes?
- When can forcible restraint be used in the emergency department?
- What constitutes sexual harassment in the workplace?
- Who should decide if an adult is incompetent?
- The meaning of suffering: a multicultural perspective.
- The Sue Rodriguez aftermath: should physicians be licensed to assist suicide?
- How does one cope with moral distress in the intensive care unit?
- Rationing and futility in the health care system.
- Is it okay to date a patient whom one likes?
- Are MDs too close to the pharmaceutical industry? Do they have conflicting interests?
- Who should know about helping patients compose an advance directive?

These sessions, each of which was usually introduced with a controversial case, worked out well and it was gratifying to see the interchange between nurses and physicians. The nurse brought his or her emphasis on the humanity of caring to counter the physician's tendency to concentrate on medical science aspects of a situation. (I had tried, but failed, to get nursing students and medical students to be taught ethics in the same classroom, though this was one of the intentions when setting up the Joint-Faculties Bioethics Project. It seemed to be a scheduling impossibility.)

THE BIOETHICS BULLETIN

In addition to the clinical and educational activities, we also saw the need to provide an avenue for publishing articles on health ethics and health law, and raising awareness of bioethics issues in health care. Thus, *The Bioethics Bulletin* began publishing about four times a year in 1989, and changed its name in 1999 to *Health Ethics Today* (see list of issues on page 182). Initially, it was distributed to all members of faculty and made available to students; later was mailed to all members of the Canadian Bioethics Society. All for free. The Faculty of Medicine paid the couple of hundred dollars each issue cost.

TABLE OF CONTENTS FOR ISSUES OF
THE BIOETHICS BULLETIN *PUBLISHED IN 1990*

Vangie Bergum, PhD, a professor of nursing and my principle associate in the ethics centre, and I had long-term plans to develop a masters program in health ethics, and as an initial step developed a graduate course in health ethics that we began offering in 1990. This became very popular, but was also hard work. We limited enrolment to 25 graduate students and offered a 13-week course—initially once annually, later twice. The most-represented faculty was nursing, but students from other health disciplines, including medicine, dentistry, pharmacy, rehabilitation and speech pathology, also enrolled. The pattern was to study an advanced bioethics text, deal with a chapter or two each week, and illustrate the topic with a video or some other method of presentation to get it on the floor for discussion.

As the course progressed, the evenings were gradually taken over by presentations from small groups of students. At the end of the course, each student submitted an essay dealing with the principle ethics issues that they faced in their work. These graduates, who had ten to 15 years of experience in health care and were very committed, were a delight to be with and to learn from. Two volumes were printed of their work.[99,100]

It is possible that a masters program in health ethics will eventually evolve from this course, but to achieve that, we need more committed ethicists, closer ties with health law, more contact with like initiatives in other Canadian universities, and more funding.

Ethics in the specialities of medicine

Apart from teaching students, I also felt my physician colleagues might benefit from our knowledge. I had some concerns about putting myself forward as a spokesman for ethics, especially in disciplines other than nephrology and transplantation. I was also concerned that my colleagues would expect me to come up with answers for some of their problems. We soon learned, however, that I had no solutions, only new ways of asking old questions and leading discussions about them. This, I came to realize, could be called "a secular casuistic approach." It bases one's ethical reasoning on (a) the true facts and circumstances of each case, and then (b) decides who are the relevant people in the relationships involved, then (c) reasons, using the relevant ethical principles, before (d) coming to a non-binding conclusion, which one (e) applies to the case. Last, one then (f) looks for the effects of applying one's conclusion to see if it holds up, or whether it needs modification. If that is indicated, then the process is cycled through again.

This approach served to make me welcome in many different clinical speciality areas, where "ethics rounds" were used to introduce dilemmas at the clinical teaching level, with residents, specialists and speciality nurses all present. The process proved to be very instructive and challenging for me. It also allowed for an educational opportunity that is not possible when doing an actual ethics bedside consultation.

Later, towards the end of my time, the Royal College in Ottawa mandated exposure to ethics in every speciality training program—all 36 of them. This greatly helped the growth of ethics teaching at the graduate level, even though no new resources were provided to meet these new obligations.

The problem in bioethics was funding

The Joint-Faculties Bioethics Project had many opportunities and was generally welcomed but, because it was not a department, or even a division of a department, there seemed to be no method of budgeting for its activities except through the discretionary funds available to the Dean. This worked for seven years without too much trouble. During the first four years, there was a supplemental budget available from an unusual source: the HLA paternity fund. This fund consisted of the earnings from an activity that I had agreed to start at the Alberta government's request several years before leaving transplantation immunology. The Department of Social Services asked us to use the tissue typing laboratory to determine fatherhood in cases of disputed paternity when the single mother applied for government assistance. The mother was asked to name a father and if that man then disputed his responsibility, he was asked to undergo blood testing for the factors of the HLA system. If this proved him to be the father, he was then asked to contribute to the upkeep of the child. It also meant that the mother was eligible for government assistance. I never quite understood what happened if he refused to be tested, or if he refused to help after paternity was established, but that was not our business. I was responsible for setting up this service and we agreed that the earnings from this activity should be placed in a trust fund for use in various ways, but should certainly not end up in anyone's professional pocket.

For the first four years after my transition into health ethics, I continued to interpret the results of this laboratory testing, including appearing in Family Court from time to time to testify about the meaning of the tests, predictability, etc. The earnings from this were used to support the field of health ethics.

After that time, my successor at the Transplant Immunology Laboratory decided to take over the funds, since the work was being done in his laboratory. He, of course, was completely entitled to do this; it was part of his responsibility and it was gracious of him not to have wanted to control the fund from the outset of his term. The technology soon changed to DNA typing anyway, which was even more definitive than HLA antigen determination of paternity and was carried out by a police laboratory. So that goose stopped laying golden eggs. A year or so later, the Joint-Faculties Bioethics Project became the Division of Bioethics, replete with a budget from the Dean of Medicine. Eventually, it became known as the John Dossetor Health Ethics Centre.

In these ways, the new thrust in health ethics grew from shaky beginnings to become an accepted element in the faculties of medicine and nursing (and to a lesser extent, in pharmacy and dentistry) and an accepted program at the University of Alberta Hospital. I felt very rewarded!

Ours was not the first bioethics program in Canada. Others were developing concurrently at Canada's 16 medical schools in various ways, largely depending on who initiated the programs. At McGill University, it was Margaret Somerville (law); at the University of Montreal, David Roy; and at the University of Toronto, Bernard Dickens (health lawyer), then Dr. Peter Singer, who built up a large group of clinicians, philosophers and lawyers. At the University of Western Ontario, the leaders were three philosophers; similarly, the University of British Columbia's Centre of Applied Ethics (Dr. Michael McDonald) is in the Department of Philosophy.

If one was to make a priority claim for the University of Alberta program, it would be on the basis of it being clinically oriented, with physicians and nurses predominating, and on being fully integrated into the medical and nursing teaching curriculum, and not being a curriculum "block" called something like Ethics and Law. We wanted ethics to become a part of clinical practice and research, and felt the best way to achieve this was by making it as applicable and accessible as possible.

Through my professional experiences, research, reading and teaching, I have become most familiar with three aspects of bioethics: clinical ethics, ethics for research on humans and transplantation relationships. The next three chapters deal with these aspects, the evolution of which followed the evolution of medicine itself, weaving a web of values en route.

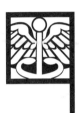

The web of our life is of a mingled yarn, good and
ill together: our virtues would be proud if our
faults whipped them not; and our crimes would
despair, if they were not cherished by our virtues.

William Shakespeare
All's Well that Ends Well (Act 4, scene 3)

Clinical ethics: Committees and consultations, 1985–1995

As MEDICAL SCIENCE PROGRESSED, bringing with it myriad lifesaving or -prolonging pharmaceuticals and revolutionary biotechnology, clinical ethics have become increasingly complex. To really appreciate this, one need only consider that before the end of World War II, medical ethics and medical etiquette were seen as part of that cherished relationship between doctor and patient, and physicians were expected to learn ethical conduct from their mentors through an apprentice system. At that time, medical knowledge was also limited. Physicians had limited means to eradicate disease by surgically removing diseased tissue. Medical understanding of disturbed physiology (the pathophysiology of disease) was rudimentary and, apart from morphine (and some of its derivatives), digitalis, vitamin C for scurvy and vitamin D for rickets, the therapeutic armamentarium was sparse indeed. The principles of the bacterial causes of infections were established and their epidemic spread was no longer attributed to the weather or to acts of fate, but there were no antibiotics. Tuberculosis was rife. On the other hand, prevention of infectious diseases through immunization and vaccination was well established and represented an enormous advance in the control of measles, diphtheria, pertussis (whooping cough), and rubella—though the differentiation of viruses, bacteria, spirochetes, fungal and rickettsia was still unknown.

Thus, much of medical care was devoted to protection, adaptation, avoidance, and acceptance and palliation of the little understood, but myriad, processes of disease. Much disease was, and still is, self-limited and of short duration. Medical reputations have long depended on the intrinsic healing power of nature. Other diseases were progressive, but could be modified somewhat. Only few disorders could be cured by medical intervention.

New roles for patients and caregivers

As medical knowledge increased, the relationship between patients and their caregivers changed. Medical knowledge was so limited before World War II that most physicians could grasp a high percentage of it. Thus, patients had reason to trust that their physicians were as well-informed as they could be, and the reputation of the profession—apart from its propensity for high fees and living well—was largely above reproach.

This is no longer true. No one can now presume to *know it all*. No physician is confident in the plenitude of his or her knowledge, even in areas of special interest. Interdependency on technology and other expertise is widespread—to the point of distancing the primary caregivers from people in need. Thus, in making clinical decisions, there are many people now at the bedside, including, most importantly, the patient who is present in a way that was relatively uncommon heretofore. Previously, the patient was expected to play a relatively passive role; after all, doctor knows best! Nowadays, in addition to the joint partnership of the patient with the medical team, including the nurse and nurse specialist, one finds the family (parents, in the case of small children, spouses and other siblings), other consultants (sometimes too many), the surrogate decision-maker (in special circumstances), the ethicist, the hospital ombudsman and the chaplain. And legal advice is always available, too. One can only hope that someone can put it all together.

The distancing effect, referred to above, is serious. Family physicians no longer visit people in their own homes. No longer is there a feeling that, when something acute happens, there will be someone you know—and who knows you—looking after you. Regrettably, we now all live, in large part, where acute and subacute situations involve strangers caring for strangers. This is much to be regretted, even though we now see that it was inevitable.

Indeed, the situation is so changed that the word "patient" should probably fade out of the medical vocabulary altogether. The word comes from the present participle of a Latin word (*patio* = *to suffer or bear a burden*). It implies suffering, but it also connotes passivity, dependency, and submissiveness. This was brought home to me quite dramatically when trying to co-ordinate a multidiscipline book called *A Handbook of*

Health Ethics in 1997.[101] We all wanted to write a book that was equally relevant to physicians, medical students, nurses, long-term care staff, physiotherapists, social workers, and others. Friendly discussion led to the possibility of several versions of the same text, using "patients" in one, "clients" in another, "residents" in another; there were some in favour of "consumers" (as in public health). It was a curious semantic impasse. In the end, sanity—or, dare I say, ethics—prevailed and we agreed to address the potential recipients of health care in its various manifestations as "people," or "individuals with...", or "people in..." Then, we hoped, a single version of the book would suffice for all. It worked, and was a lesson to me in consensus building and in new ways of showing respect for others' dignity.

The pace of biotechnology

Nowadays the complexity of medical ethics is growing exponentially with rapid advances in biotechnology. Each year, there are new questions of profound significance that probe at the basis and origin of life, including, for example, ectogenesis (the artificial womb); xenotransplantation (using animal organs for transplant of vital organs); issues of wrongful birth (children suing parents for giving birth to them, knowing the fetus to have conditions that would make them suffer); preserving stem cells from the umbilical cord blood for possible later use by that newborn; obtaining embryonic stem cells from surplus embryos (surplus from procedures used *in vitro* fertilizations; the right not to be resuscitated after cardiopulmonary arrest.

In these newer areas of the health ethics debate, agreement on language and definition of terms becomes important. This is especially true in discussing the ethics of human development. Thus:

- *zygote* denotes the earliest product of human conception, prior to cell divisions;
- *blastocyst:* the pre-embryo at five to seven days, with approximately 100 cells, called *blastomeres*, with an inner cell mass from which stems cells can be grown and from which the fetus will develop, and an outer coat of cells—the *trophoblast*—which develop into the placenta;
- *pre-embryo* denotes development from conception to 14 days, at which time the primitive streak appears and twinning is

no longer possible. Some international research legislation limits development *in vitro* to this 14-day pre-embryo period;

- *embryo* denotes development from zygote stage to nine weeks, by which time all rudimentary organs are present, including the neural tube. The term includes blastocyst and pre-embryo stages;
- *fetus* applies from about nine weeks (the neural tube denoting the beginnings of formation of the brain) to full term;
- *person* (probably the most controversial of all) means, in the context of the law, the personal legal rights attributed only to those who have been born and exist independently, but ethics does not necessarily offer such a clear definition.

Similar definitions are needed for other discussion areas. In the ethics of end-of-life situations, it is critical to define such concepts as "withholding treatment" *versus* "withdrawing treatment," "life prolonging" *versus* "prolonging dying," "life support that can give benefit" *versus* "life support that cannot give benefit" (to the person whose life is under consideration), "harms of primary intention" *versus* "unavoidable but unintended, indirect harm," "passive euthanasia" *versus* "allowing to die." And the list goes on.

Central to all these issues is the process by which individuals make decisions based on "informed consent" (though, as stated earlier, I much prefer the concept to of "comprehended choice," in which the legal standard of "what a reasonable person needs to know" is replaced by "what a reasonable person has clearly understood").

Table 11.1 lists some of the milestones that have led to the recent evolutionary stages of health ethics at the individual level. Thus, Table 11.1 might be taken to illustrate the fleshing out of the three bioethics mantras:

1. respecting and promoting autonomy,
2. beneficence (do good), and
3. non-malfeasance (do no harm).

Table 11.1 might be taken as the fourth Georgetown mantra: distributive justice or fairness in the delivery systems for health care.

A quick glance at Table 11.1 shows that life and death issues—the big-ticket items of clinical ethics—predominate. I have grouped these milestones together by topic: nephrology, transplantation, neonatology, abortion and end-of-life issues, many of which took place in the U.S. (The

Table 11.1 Milestones of health ethics.

Year	Practice Area	Example
1962/63	Nephrology	The Seattle nephrology group (Scribner) seeks help in selection of people with chronic renal failure for long-term maintenance hemodialysis
1963	Transplantation	Cadaveric organ transplantation starts
1966	Clinical research	Henry Beecher's exposure of informed consent and other issues in academic research published in the *New England Journal of Medicine*
1968	Transplantation	First heart transplant (performed by C. Barnard)
1968	Transplantation	Definition of brain death by Harvard Committee[102]
1969	Neonatology	Down's syndrome baby allowed to die at Johns Hopkins
1971	Neonatology	Three-day conference, "Human Rights, Retardation & Research," leads to formation of Kennedy Institute of Ethics at Georgetown
1973	Neonatology	R.S. Duff, Alistair Campbell: "Moral & ethical dilemmas in the special-care nursery"[103]
1975	Neonatology	AR Jonsen: "Critical Issues in Newborn Intensive Care: Conference and Policy Proposal"[104]
1982	Neonatology	Baby Doe led to U.S. federal government regulations which were abandoned after challenge from Society of Pediatrics
1973	Abortion (U.S.)	U.S. Supreme Court: *Roe v Wade*
1988	Abortion (Canada)	Abortion struck from the Criminal Code of Canada as unconstitutional
1976	End of life	Karen Quinlan case decided (New Jersey Supreme Court): family allowed to discontinue her respirator in her vegetative state. She lived nine more years.
1976	End of life	Mass. General Hospital forms ethics committee to decide on "Optimal care of hopelessly ill patients"[105]
1976	End of life	C. Fried: "Terminating Life Support: Out of the Closet"[106]
1976	End of life	The birth of the living will and advance directives; S. Bok: "Personal Decisions for care at the end of life"[107]
1978	End of life	A. Relman: "The Saikewicz Decision: Judges as Physicians"[108]
1986	End of life	R. Steinbrook, B. Lo: "Artificial Feeding—Solid Ground, Not a Slippery Slope";[109] The Brophy case: withdrawal of food and fluid, in persistent vegetative states
1986	End of life	Holland permits active euthanasia under strict rules
1990	End of life	M. Angell: "Prisoner of Technology—Nancy Cruzan"[110] Cruzan case defines levels of decision-making for incompetent adults
1991	End of life (Canada)	Nancy B. (25 years old, paralysis, mentally alert) seeks discontinuation of therapy with ventilator. Court eventually grants her wish and she dies.[111]
1993	End of life (Canada)	Sue Rodriguez denied assistance in suicide by Supreme Court of Canada (5–4 split) but it happens anyway[112]
1980	Standard of information disclosure (Canada)	*Reibl v. Hughes* [1980] 2 SCR 880. MDs must disclose what "a reasonable person in the patient's position" might need to know

issues of clinical research are dealt with in Chapter 12, and are seldom issues of life and death. I return to transplant ethics in Chapter 13.)

Ethical dilemmas in neonatology illustrate how delicately balanced these issues are and how difficult they are to resolve. Should one try to preserve children with gross developmental defects? If not, who decides who should live? Are parents, who have the ongoing responsibility for care, not crucial to that ethical decision? If so, how does one give them enough information in situations of great uncertainty? Should surgery be offered to all children born with spina bifida? Can these decisions be regulated by government, as tried for a period in 1982–1983, when the Reagan administration in the U.S. instituted a government hotline for reporting severely handicapped newborns whom someone suspected would be neglected by physicians? Should all the stops be pulled out for premature children who weigh less than one kilogram at birth? How about half a kilogram? In my view, every neonatologist is a clinical ethicist of great experience, but no one envies this difficult aspect of their work.

Similar agonies have been experienced by those trying to make the "ought" decisions at the end of adult life. Most of these milestones needed a court decision to resolve them. More often than not, it was the family that took the institution and its physicians to court. From these judgements, family decisions and advanced directives (living wills) have usually prevailed over physician opinions. In the wake of these decisions, the previous paternalism lies mauled beyond hope of recovery, but a new relationship has emerged that integrates decision-making of the family, the expressed opinion of the person concerned (directly, or through advance directives or surrogate decision makers) and caregivers. This is a large step towards "comprehended choice."

In the case of Karen Quinlan, the highly publicized case of a young woman in a persistent vegetative state (PVS), the family successfully persuaded a New Jersey Superior Court to allow a life-sustaining respirator to be removed in the clear expectation of her death. In fact, she breathed just enough to maintain life and lingered in a PVS for another nine years without any perception or return of consciousness.

Paul Brophy, a 47-year-old firefighter who entered the PVS after brain surgery, was maintained by stomach tube feedings, though he did not need a ventilator. A year or so later, his wife and family petitioned to have the food and fluid stopped and the tube into his stomach removed. Their will was granted by a court against the will of the physicians and hospital. This was the first case in which it was judged that there were circumstances where food and fluid could be stopped because no benefit was being conferred. Later, there was a similar judgement in U.K. by the House of Lords for a young man, Anthony Bland, aged 17 when injured, who had been in a PVS for five years.[113]

In Canada, there have been two precedent-setting instances involving end-of-life decisions, Nancy B. in Quebec and Sue Rodriguez in British Columbia, because both had *full mental competence*. Nancy B., 25, suffered from irrecoverable but no longer progressive Guillain-Barre paralysis. She sought action through her lawyer for a court to order the physician and hospital to turn off the respirator on which she was totally dependent. She obtained her wish and died. In contrast, however, Sue Rodriguez, also fully competent and mentally alert, wanted the Supreme Court of Canada to sanction her desire to have her physician assist her suicide at the time when she wanted it (she had not reached the point of being ventilator-dependent). The Supreme Court denied this wish by a split vote (5–4), though this is what subsequently is presumed to have happened when she died shortly thereafter.

The case of Nancy Cruzan, a young American woman in a PVS, is notable in that the U.S. Supreme Court acknowledged three levels of decision-making: the *subjective* level (where an incompetent person has left clear and convincing evidence of what they might want to happen to them, such as in a living will); the *substituted judgement* level (where others had evidence of the person's wishes from statements and conversations, but nothing was in writing), and the *best interests* level (where judgements are made by third parties who try to decide what the person would have decided and what action would be in his/her best interest). These degrees of decision-making are very useful guidelines in difficult situations.

In this series of cases, end-of-life court decisions were made for people who:

- were mentally incompetent and respirator dependent, *or*
- were incompetent but not respirator-dependent, but maintained by artificially-administered food and fluid, *with or without* having left "clear and convincing" evidence of their wishes for such circumstances, *or*
- were fully competent people who did not wish to be kept alive by others when it was impossible to recover to what

they considered to be a minimally acceptable quality of life
(Nancy B.), *or*

- wished to have help bringing about their own demise when
  they lacked physical capacity to effect this for themselves
  (Sue Rodriguez).

Institutional Ethics Committees

Taking such actions to court was against all the traditions of medical
practice and was bitterly resented by some. There is now general
agreement that the courts are not the best places to make such difficult
decisions. The preferred route is now the Institutional Ethics Committee
(IEC), Clinical Ethics Consultative Committees, or Medical Moral
Committees, which have become very widespread since 1983. These
committees are comprised of physicians, pastoral care people, social
service personnel, nurses, dieticians, neonatology nurses, and one or more
members of the public-at-large. They are closer to the scene, but not close
enough to become emotionally involved in the actual decision-making.
They can learn details of the dilemma and consider pertinent research
and discuss and ponder solutions in ways that are not possible by justices
in a court.

These committees—I use the term Institutional Ethics Committee—
may be seen as a spin-off of the committees that reviewed ethics in
clinical research protocols. These research committees, known in the U.S.
as Institutional Research Boards (IRBs) and in Canada as Research Ethics
Boards (REBs), are discussed in Chapter 12; the roles of these two
committees are quite different from IECs.

The IECs, which report to institutions such as hospitals or regional
health groupings, should play an important role in drafting institutional
policy. Ethics situations arising at the bedside may be dealt with by the
IEC, by local discussion groups, or by consulting with others who might
be able to bring a different perspective to the situation. There are no
official provincial or national agencies for accreditation or evaluation of
IECs. Indeed, formal accreditation procedures do not exist for REBs either,
but the funding agencies are able to exert influence on the quality of ethics
review for research. No external agency plays a similar role for IECs.

Despite its unofficial status, clinical ethics involvement (consultant,
local discussion, or IEC) has come to be a significant factor in contemporary
clinical encounters. The reader will have to judge whether they are likely

to be sufficient to stem the effect of lessened trust and impaired relationship between those who receive care and those who provide it.

This erosion of trust is due to such factors as:

- the distancing effect of new technologies;
- the "tyranny of the white coat" and the absence of house calls;
- the increased number of care providers in the management team;
- the increased specialization of consultant physicians;
- the enormous increase in knowledge and of possible options for action, some of which can cause harm;
- the duty rotations of physicians in hospitals (month on month off, etc.). In some parts of a modern hospital many patients cannot name the physician who is looking after them; in some areas, they form a majority;
- the 5:00 p.m. evening and weekend sign-off for family practitioners, suggesting the use of walk-in clinics or local emergency rooms for off-hour problems;
- the increased sources available to individuals to learn about their illnesses for themselves;
- the tendency for litigation when allegedly harmed in some way.

Many of these factors are valid reasons why house calls will never become the norm again for family practice, even though there are technologies that might make a partial return possible. Still, people are so different when one sees them in their homes, where the visiting physician is a guest. Let us hope that we will never let go entirely of this ideal.

All these factors, and the milestone events that preceded them, are the reasons ethics has become such a widely discussed aspect of contemporary health care, and will surely increase in the future. The professional who goes into ethics can expect to be involved in consultations on difficult problems, to be asked to serve on both IECs and REBs, and to undertake interdisciplinary educational discussions: bioethics rounds. These have now become the daily bread of ethics personnel, including myself after 1985.

Milestones of health policy

Underlying the medical aspects of bioethics are public policy factors that have also contributed to the increasing importance of ethics in health care. Public policy draws its ethical principle from the *fourth* Georgetown mantra of *Distributive Justice*.[114]

In much of the Western world, though to a lesser degree in the U.S., society has decided that concern for the health of its citizens should be a responsibility of governments. This has led to the introduction of publicly funded health services *at the individual level* and through *collective public health* services (vaccination and immunization programs, programs for clean water and effective sewage disposal, etc.).

Table 11.2 highlights some of the main events in the evolution of publicly funded health services. All these initiatives came after World War II, beginning in the town of Swift Current, Saskatchewan, which was the first in North America to have a public insurance program for health, making health services available to all residents in that town in 1946. Britain introduced a National Health Service in 1948.

In most countries, medical professional organizations vigorously opposed the introduction of universal health insurance. The fear was that the government would destroy professional autonomy, make every physician a government employee and stifle initiative. But for individual physicians—distinct from the collective opinions of the more politically-oriented colleges and associations—these measures have been applauded and embraced. Nowadays, the colleges and associations, as well as many individual physicians, defend these principles when they are threatened by interests (including governments hoping to save money or private for-profit entrepreneurs) that seek to turn health care back to the market place, with adequate care going to the wealthy, but not, necessarily, to those in most need. Indeed, maintaining the principles of the *Canada Health Act*, which most Canadians warmly embrace, has become a highly charged political and ethical debate.

This is not the place for an extended discussion of the issues involved, such as rising costs, increasing technologies, the need for reform of services (less in-hospital care, more community and home care), the effect of the ageing population and enormous increases in drug costs. Only the future will reveal how Canadians will get health care. Most now want it to remain in the public arena, and many even want coverage to be extended to drug costs (pharmacare) and want home care. It remains the chief political issue in Canada, even in the age of terrorism.

Table 11.2 Individual health services—publicly funded.

1946	Swift Current, Saskatchewan, introduces public insurance.
1948	U.K.: Birth of the National Health Service.
1962	Saskatchewan: Tommy Douglas introduces Medicare.
1966	U.S. introduces Medicare for all citizens over 65 and Medicaid for the indigent and the working poor. All others are insured through employers or private insurance, if at all (in 2000, some 45 million people lacked any health insurance).
1966	Canada's National Medicare Bill (227) is approved, with the federal government paying 50 per cent of federal, provincial and territorial health care costs.
1972	U.S. Congress extends Medicaid coverage to all age groups with end-stage renal disease (dialysis and renal transplantation).
1983	U.K., Prime Minister Margaret Thatcher introduces two-tiered individual health care.
1984	*Canada Health Act* introduced with 5 principles: public funding; universal coverage of all people; comprehensive service coverage; accessibility for all; interprovincial portability.
2000	Alberta's Bill 11 (Ralph Klein) opens the door to private for-profit surgical facilities.
	Roy Romanow produces a report entitled Future of Health Care in Canada.
	Members to the new Canadian Health Council are appointed.

Experiences of a clinical ethics consultant

Not long after the formation of the Joint-Faculties Bioethics Project in 1986, I was asked to become involved in some clinical situations with dominant ethics issues. Many of these were related to end-of-life issues, and it was with some diffidence—stemming from a feeling of inadequacy—that I explored them with those who were directly and often emotionally involved. In some situations, I was personally asked to carry out an ethics consultation; in others, I was invited in my capacity as chairperson of the IEC at the University of Alberta Hospital. In both types of situation, I preferred to take a nurse and one other health professional with me, though I wrote the consultation note myself. The steps involved in the process of an ethical consultation are shown in Figure 11.1.

There are some concerns about ethics consultations that I have never fully resolved. What is one's legal status when doing one? Does the medical protective insurance, which all physicians carry, cover those acting in an ethics consultative capacity outside the context of their recognized medical speciality? What is one's legal liability when offering advice or opinions that might then, because the future is always unpredictable, turn out to lead to some sort of harm? It is because of these sorts of concerns that most IECs do not actually recommend solutions to problems. Rather, they document opinions, analyze situations from an

Figure 11.1 The ethical consultation process.

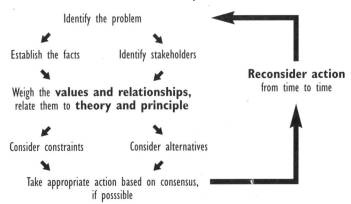

Identify the problem

Establish the facts   Identify stakeholders

Weigh the **values and relationships**, relate them to **theory and principle**

Consider constraints   Consider alternatives

Take appropriate action based on consensus, if posssible

Reconsider action from time to time

ethical perspective, document ethical flaws in different positions, and, most importantly, talk to all parties on the assumption that all are acting in good faith in the search for the best outcome.

The following are some examples of the end-of-life problems I have encountered (all altered to preserve confidentiality). In recording these examples, I do not claim that they describe the range of ethics consultations or paint an accurate picture of the consultant's professional life. The examples are taken from memory and presented here to give a picture of the sort of involvement in ethics that I found to be my lot.

A woman with amyotrophic lateral sclerosis who refused to drink

L.P., a 54-year-old woman, had progressive amyotrophic lateral sclerosis (ALS or Lou Gherig's disease), a degenerative condition of the spinal cord that does not affect the brain directly. People with this condition remain competent and alert while progressively suffering from weakness, immobility, limb wasting and in the later stages, have difficulty swallowing and coughing. Eventually they choke to death or die of pneumonia. In Canada, Sue Rodriguez was a well-known example of someone suffering from this condition.

L.P., who was in a long-term care hospital, was not an easy patient. She proved testy with the staff and was difficult with her husband; as a result, their relationship was very strained. She had an acerbic attitude despite her dependence on others. She also lived through the media-soaked end of Sue Rodriguez's life, but L.P. decided on another course.

When she deemed the time had come, she made clear her wish that she would stop eating and taking fluids with a view to inducing her own death. She wanted reassurance from the staff that they would not give her fluids intravenously or by subdermal clysis (running in fluid slowly under soft areas of skin), or force her to take food by mouth, stomach tube, or percutaneous gastrostomy—a relatively easy tube puncture through the abdominal wall to the outside from within the stomach, using a gastroscope. This tube can then be used to place food and fluids into the stomach directly.

Would agreeing to her request be assisting suicide? If so, it is against the Criminal Code of Canada (sections 14[*] and 241[§]). Would agreeing be tantamount to denying the *care* that every hospital is obliged to give? The Code states that if anyone who has the obligation of care fails to give that care and this subsequently leads to another's death, then a crime has been committed (sections 215[†] and 217[‡]).

I became involved in the case of L.P. at the request of the administration and the nursing staff, though I also made contact with the responsible physician and made sure that he knew of my pending involvement, and, later, my view of the matter. I met L.P. and was convinced that she was competent. This being so, her autonomy should prevail. In my view, they

---

[*] No person is entitled to consent to have death inflicted upon him, and such consent does not affect the criminal responsibility of any person by whom death may be inflicted upon the person by whom consent is given.

[§] Every one who (a) counsels a person to commit suicide, or (b) aids or abets a person to commit suicide, whether suicide ensues or not, is guilty of an indictable offence and is liable to imprisonment for a term not exceeding 14 years (*Sections of the Criminal Code of Canada*).

[†] (1) Everyone is under a legal duty...to provide necessaries of life to a person under his charge if that person

    (i)   is unable, by reason of detention, age, illness, mental disorder or other cause, to withdraw himself from that charge, and

    (ii) is unable to provide himself with necessaries of life....

  (2) Every one commits an offence who, being under a legal duty within the meaning of subsection (1), fails...to perform that duty, if...with respect to a duty imposed by paragraph (1)(c), the failure to perform the duty endangers the life of the person to whom the duty is owed...is guilty of (a) an indictable offence and is liable to imprisonment for a term not exceeding two years; or (b) an offence punishable on summary conviction.

[‡] Duty of persons undertaking acts: every one who undertakes to do an act is under a legal duty to do it if an omission to do the act is or may be dangerous to life.

were not actively assisting her to die, and would not be justified in overruling her autonomy to prevent her from dying in the way she had chosen. She died in a week (of dehydration, not starvation). The only treatment given was to keep moist the mucous membranes of her mouth and pharynx. Her death was not agonizing. She did not complain of thirst—reminding me of when I had been a guinea pig in a dehydration experiment at McGill in the late 1950s and had discovered that depriving a person of all fluid leads to raging thirst is false; in fact, the urgent sense of thirst goes after 24 to 26 hours.

The peaceful way in which L.P. died emphasized to me that other health professionals should know that this is a way of allowing death to close an overburdened life when that life can no longer bring benefit. In her last days, L.P. re-established good relationships with her family and the hospital staff, several of the latter coming in on their days off be with her as the end approached. She had control, and this gave L.P. real satisfaction, a state which became evident to others. The process was so much better than physician-assisted suicide or voluntary active euthanasia would have been.[115] There was an element of closure and acceptance when she died.

The man whose family insisted on repeated attempts at CPR
Another end-of-life consultation concerned a 65-year-old man, C.D., who had renal failure and had been on hemodialysis for 18 months. One day he had a sudden myocardial infarction after a dialysis treatment. While in the coronary care unit, he had a cardiac arrest and was immediately resuscitated. Despite some recovery of heart function, he remained unconscious and unrousable, had stopped breathing on his own and required a mechanical ventilator. His cardiac status did not become stable. It seemed that the heart could not sustain adequate blood flow and he had a subsequent cardiac arrest. Again he was resuscitated and again the subsequent heart status was very unstable. He failed to show any signs of consciousness (no spontaneous breathing, no response to pain). Was he alive? One certainly could not say he was dead. One might speculate that these two periods of cardiac standstill, at his age, would cause very serious damage to the brain and provide a very poor outlook for brain function if he survived.

After the third resuscitation, at the end of the second day, the physician advised the family that C.D. would never have adequate brain function if he survived, although he probably was not brain dead. By this time, his son had arrived from San Diego. He had missed the first 24 hours of this episode and, indeed, had not seen his father for some years. He confronted the physician and insisted that further resuscitation must take place if cardiac arrest reoccurred. The physician performed this twice more and then consulted the hospital administration, who supported the son's point of view, even though this view was not shared by C.D.'s daughter or wife. All this happened between Christmas and New Year's, when normal deliberation and full consultation is difficult, but an ethics consultation was requested by the physician and I became involved.

By the time I entered the situation, two more resuscitations had taken place and it was clear that there would be no recovery. The real problem was the son's denial of the inevitable outcome. I thought that the only worthwhile treatment objective was to help the son adjust to reality, even if it meant continuing with resuscitations for a while longer and enduring abuse from the staff who wanted it resolved quickly. The chaplain agreed to sit with the family to try to get close to the son.

There is no right way to handle such a situation. It does not come from a book, it comes from humans interacting under difficult situations in efforts to empower their human relationships. In addition to staff abuse, the situation was also using a lot of resources. After two more efforts at resuscitation, the son said he could not take it any more and asked that further treatment be stopped. His father was then declared dead. I was particularly grateful to the chaplain.

This case illustrates how difficult these situations are, and how impossible it is to decide on first principles. From the principle viewpoint, the prognosis was hopeless after the second of seven resuscitations. From that time point on, acceptable recovery of brain activity would not occur and many would therefore say further treatment was futile. In that event, one would have been justified in refusing any more cardiopulmonary resuscitation (CPR), even though no one could say that full and complete death of the brain and brain stem—the definition of brain death—had taken place. C.D.'s wife and daughter were ready to accept that CPR was futile, but the son was not. This is an excellent example of how ethics and relationships are intertwined.

In my view, it said a lot for the sensitivity of the treating physician that she was able to consider the son's viewpoint and, together with the staff, help the son cope with an unacceptable situation. But was the physician abusing the father—in futile therapy—to accommodate the grieving process of the son? Quite possibly. But then, was the father feeling anything at all? No, certainly not. He had been totally and deeply unconscious for several days. Did the ethicist help? Probably not, except to support those who could see past the medical exigencies and try to cope with the meaning of this human tragedy to those involved.

There are many speculative aspects of these tragic few days in the life of that family and the hospital staff. It is impossible to analyze and answer all the questions. But that is how ethical dilemmas often run. It says something that the family was satisfied with the way things were handled and expressed gratitude to the staff (see also an excellent paper on "Distant and Close-Up Ethics"[116]).

A young woman with severe mental disability and breasts that impaired breathing

Until 1971, Alberta legislation permitted a committee to decide whether a mentally disabled person should be sterilized. The Act had been passed 40 years before, when it was believed that mental disability was congenital and could be passed on. It was the age of social eugenics designed to theoretically build a "better" population of Albertans. Such measures were fairly widespread before World War II, after which they were exposed and condemned following the atrocities in Nazi Germany when thousands of acts of barbarity were committed against mentally disabled people—prior to the systematic extermination of certain ethnic groups, especially the Jews. These heinous acts are felt by all those charged with making decisions for the mentally disabled today.

This historical background caused much discussion and soul-searching over the problems that beset P.M., a 32-year-old woman who had been mentally disabled since birth, had never been able to speak but was able to express emotions of appreciation for her mother and care providers (especially nurses). At the time of this consultation, the mother was 65 and concerned about her daughter's future. She had been appointed by a court as P.M.'s legal guardian many years earlier.

P.M. was unable to walk, but could be placed in a wheelchair. She seemed to be sensitive to music and sunshine. She also liked to eat, which is where the problem arose. She gained considerable weight and mammary development became so great that her breasts became an impediment to breathing at night if she rolled onto her back. Obviously the nurses would try to help her avoid this problem, though P.M. had no insight into what caused her to waken in a panicked state during the night. Nor did she have enough strength to turn herself over once she had rolled onto her back.

Her mother requested breast reduction surgery. The plastic surgeon was concerned that such surgery would be seen as being done mainly for the benefit of care providers and P.M.'s mother, and not P.M. herself. The breasts were not the site of pathology; they were normal, just very large. He suggested instituting dietary reduction. Losing 20 kilograms (44 pounds) would probably solve the problem. He wondered about the ethics of such surgery and requested an ethics opinion.

I felt that I needed time to assess everyone's degree of commitment and to form an opinion about their motives. A three-month period of serious weight reduction was instituted by the institution's dietician but had little success, largely because P.M. demanded more than she was given, and her poorly-articulated but strongly-urged demands could not be resisted. Opinions from others were obtained and her case was presented to the IEC.

In the end, after a bout of pneumonia when it was feared she would need intubation, and with further urging from her mother, breast reduction was carried out. Her situation improved immediately and remained so.

One might ask, why all the fuss? Her mother had legal decision-making authority, so why not go ahead? The answer is that life's dilemmas are not solved as simply as that. Suppose that there had been a post-operative complication, someone could easily have challenged both the mother and surgeon for involving P.M. in "unnecessary" surgery, carried out for the convenience of caregivers.

Those who have served for years on IECs are familiar with the problems related to trying to care for mentally challenged (legally incompetent) people. This is just one example. The use of restraints—physical or pharmacological—provides another. More common, perhaps, is the use of percutaneous gastrostomy tubes for feeding people who are stuporous, or similarly incompetent, and unable to feed themselves. When cared for in an active general hospital, the nursing burden for such people is great. But when the problem dictates that they should really be in a long-term or auxiliary hospital or nursing home, it is often suggested that they have a gastrostomy tube inserted directly though the abdominal wall for the convenience of those who look after them. Gastroenterologists, who are asked to insert these tubes, are usually very concerned about the ethics of such a procedure. One of them challenged the ethics centre to produce guidelines to help with such situations, and we accepted the challenge. In 1990, an ethics task force, led by nurse Donna Wilson, PhD, was established, and a number of highly informative discussions with various experts led to the publication of guidelines that were later made widely available and used in many institutions across Canada. The whole topic, and its ethics, has been the subject of a recent seminal review.[117]

C.C. and the persistent incognitive vegetative state

A very distressing situation that occurs about 200 times annually in Canada is called the persistent incognitive vegetative state (PIVS). Karen Quinlan became a world famous instance of this syndrome in the U.S. in the 1970s. I was privileged to become involved with a similar family in Edmonton after their son had sustained a serious head injury. He had been fooling around with friends one summer evening, riding on the front of a van that was careering around a vacant parking lot. Both the boy and his friend who was driving the van had been drinking. The inevitable happened when the van braked sharply and C.C. fell head first onto the pavement and sustained a severe head injury.

The neurosurgeons did what they could, but the main problem was brain swelling. This so impaired brain blood flow (due to rise of pressure within the rigid skull) that a great deal of damage was done. Three weeks later he was able to breathe without assistance, but remained unconscious and totally unresponsive to painful stimuli. At three months, it was noted that his eyes were open for periods of time and he appeared to have wake and sleep periods, but he was still completely unconscious and unable to communicate in any way. Nutrition was maintained by a feeding tube through the abdominal wall directly into his stomach.

The vegetative state diagnosis cannot be made until at least six months—and some would say as long as one year. It is characterized by wake and sleep periods, associated with spontaneous breathing, "unseeing and unhearing wakeful unawareness," complete paralysis and unresponsiveness, and a destroyed cerebral cortex but preserved brain stem functions. People have survived up to 34 years in such a state.

An important philosophical question is whether they are alive or not. I will not enter into that debate here, but the family believed C.C. was alive and instituted cerebral stimulation. They put his limbs through full range of movement every hour. They organized groups of volunteers to be with him and to take him out to shopping malls in a wheelchair. This was all part of assisting C.C.'s brain to react to his environment. Of course, there was one prime mover in this enormous effort of love: his sister, L.C., who devoted most of her time to his care.

It would be wonderful if this love had paid off. I can think of two cases that seemed equally hopeless at eight weeks post-injury and where recovery occurred. In both of these cases, mental capacity at two years was really almost normal. But such was not to be the outcome for C.C.

I became involved in the fourth year of this devoted attention. I was asked by the nursing director to see him, with the agreement of the visiting physician, and with the knowledge of C.C's sister. She had gradually come to realize that there had been no change in her brother's condition even though there had also been no deterioration. She had come to doubt whether he still inhabited his own body. Had his soul left the body? This was now her main concern. This was also the concern of C.C's parents, who were devout Catholics. They had concluded that soullessness was not living. L.C. was also questioning her purpose in life. It was one thing to devote herself to her brother's eventual recovery of brain function, but quite another to spend her life looking after his soulless body. In short, she believed that the feeding tube should be removed and her brother's material body should be allowed to die.

There was no doubt in anyone's mind that she wanted his soul to return, but no longer believed it could. But who could give authority for what she now felt was the right thing to do? The physician? The family? The Church? The ethicist? Or was it simply that no one could? In discussing this with her, we concluded that authorization lay with all those who loved C.C. By this time, that included all those on the hospital staff who had looked after him over the years, as well as his family. A plan was made that any discontinuation would be done openly and with the foreknowledge of all those who loved C.C. Several meetings with the hospital staff and the family took place. Open discussion was invited concerning discontinuation of the feeding tube. There was much expression of love and understanding for L.C. as a result of this openness. It was a moving experience for everyone. A reporter from the local paper was present at the final meeting and wrote an article with deep understanding of the motives and methods.

On an agreed-upon day, the feeding tube was removed. He died in five days. Many of the staff visited him during those last days. They seemed to want to be there. Not a single person expressed moral misgivings. L.C. and other family members were present around the clock, and the staff and family became close. After C.C. died, another meeting of the family and hospital staff was held with pastoral staff and the local priest. Many of the staff also attended his funeral.

Was this ethics? Was the course an ethically appropriate one? Could someone claim that an offence was committed under the Criminal Code? In my judgement, the answer to all three questions is yes. Am I content to now write about it, confessing my own complicity in the matter? Again, affirmative!

Clinical ethics is able to reach out ahead of the law, in this and a number of other areas. I think it is the fear of moral controversy that paralyses lawmakers (and law revisionists, i.e., politicians). One must admit that the Canadian Senate Social Affairs Committee made an effort in 1997 in their review of euthanasia and physician-assisted suicide and their subsequent recommendation that Parliament consider "compassionate homicide" as a category under the Canadian Criminal Code, with a lesser penalty.[118] This was addressed by the *Canadian Medical Association Journal* in 1997,[119] but nothing was subsequently done by the government.

If C.C.'s case was an example of ethics, what principles were involved at the end? Beneficence? Yes, towards C.C., L.C., the staff, and the rest of the family. Medical futility? No, I reject the notion of futility (it is too final, too exclusive, too distancing) in favour of "inability to provide benefit." Recognition of this inability made further maintenance of tube feeding meaningless to L.C. I think the rest of his family had reached that conclusion some months earlier.

Not mentioned in this account is the question of resource use and the ability of a family to provide sufficient funding to continue care. If ever there were situations where the humanity of the Canadian health care system is demonstrated, it is with patients such as C.C. How would the course have run, and for how long, in a system where there was insufficient funding to support individuals such as C.C. over a period of many months. The answer, of course, is that he would have died as soon as the family resources were exhausted. A very important consensus of this sort of end-of-life problem came out of the Appleton consensus, which remains a great example of how ethics can work.[120] Thirty-three physicians, bioethicists, and medical economists from ten different countries met at Lawrence University in Appleton, Wisconsin, to create a consensus for four specific decision-making circumstances: (1) five guidelines, in three categories, for decisions involving competent patients or patients who have executed an advance directive before becoming incompetent; (2) thirteen guidelines for decisions involving patients who were once competent, but are not now competent, and who have not executed an advance directive; (3) seven guidelines for decisions involving patients who are not now and never have been competent, for whom "no substituted judgement" can be rendered; and (4) eleven guidelines for decisions on scarce medical resources, where five concepts were identified as critical for the establishment of priorities.

Not all the serious quality-of-life consultations lead to negative assessments. Ethics committees are not mechanisms for making decisions that lead to diminished care in order to save resources. This is illustrated by the following consultation. Again the example deals with a seriously disabled person who was in need of life-long protection.

A quality of life assessment consultation

Great devotion and self-commitment are often shown toward people with severe disabilities by those who love them. Tragically, some are abandoned by their immediate family, but others mercifully take on the task of caring for them. Below is a copy of my consultation (altered to preserve privacy) for a man who was admitted to hospital with severe dehydration and was unable to fend for himself.

The case of Walter Court on page 208 illustrates that ethics consultations must take into account many people's viewpoints. They involve physicians but are not medical decisions. It is important, of course, to keep the physicians involved by having discussions with others, independent of a semi-public meeting. The fact remains that the legal liability for most of these sorts of decisions rests with the responsible physician and not with the ethicist or the committee.

The case shows why the role of ethics is to assess and summarize the various issues and viewpoints but not to make recommendations. Recommendations by an ethics committee, if not followed, might lead to the physician being asked in a court why he or she did not follow the recommendation. This might not be wrong, but it is a process that physicians might want to avoid. Usually, as in Walter's case, the

CONSULTATION REPORT ON WALTER COURT

Thank you for asking the Ethics Committee to be involved in decisions for this 34-year-old person. Walter was admitted recently in an unconscious dehydrated state. He has had cerebral palsy since birth and mental retardation. He has some epileptic seizure activity (presumably, grand mal type). He is incontinent of bowel and bladder, though this is coped with by diapering. He has had bedsores in the past, but not at present. He is living in a group home. Has no family and is under guardianship of the Public Guardian.

The question posed was whether his quality of life was so low that treatment to stabilize his fluid and food intake by *insertion of a PEG feeding tube might not be in his best interests.*

A small group from the Ethics Committee (a nurse, a social worker, John Dossetor) met with the physicians (Drs. J., Y. and H.) and nurses in charge of Walter, plus two caregivers from the group home, Walter's guardian, and two representatives from the Public Guardian's office—about 12 persons in all. By the time of this meeting certain new facts had emerged which helped clarify the issue of Walter's quality of life. It is better than was thought, initially.

Walter is able to achieve quite a lot of interaction with his environment. This includes recognizing and bonding with people, satisfaction in some elements of life (eating, music, affection for others, affection from others, external stimulation of various sorts). He has a life plan made for his needs which lays down certain goals for living. These were not available at the time of initial assessment and it is desirable that copies of these documents be requested of the Guardian's office so that they might be available on a future admission.

After discussion, the physicians responsible for Walter, together with nurses, expressed the view that it seemed evident that Walter would derive benefit from PEG tube feeding and therefore supported the view of the Guardians and Home Caregivers. Subsequent periodic review would be appropriate. We are glad that this consensus was achieved.

consultation report compares different viewpoints and states whether one or the other can be supported as ethically appropriate and sound. But the real value of Walter's consultation came from the meeting of 12 or so minds and the discussion that enabled their consensus opinion at the end of the process.

These examples give an idea of the issues that lead to bedside consultation with a health ethicist. I have chosen to use examples with end-of-life dilemmas because those are the most common reasons for consultation in an active general hospital. Such dilemmas also include resource allocation issues, issues of autonomy, issues of quality of life, issues of assisting suicide, issues of euthanasia, and issues of decision-making for the incompetent person. However inadequate this account is of the whole field of health ethics, it provides a glimpse of the career I adopted in 1985. I believe they are examples of secular casuistry in action.

Two special fields remain: the *ethics issues of clinical researchs* and the complex *ethics issues of organ transplantation*. The next two chapters will deal with these areas.

Know then thyself, presume not God to scan;
The proper study of mankind is man.

———————

Plac'd on this isthmus of a middle state,
A being, darkly wise and rudely great:
With too much knowledge for the sceptic side,
With too much weakness for the stoic's pride,
He hangs between; in doubt to act, or rest; …
Alike in ignorance, his reason such,
Whether he thinks too little, or too much:
Sole judge of truth, in endless error hurl'd:
The glory, jest, and riddle of the world! …

———————

Go, wondrous creature! mount where science guides,
Go, measure earth, weigh air, and state the tides;
For Reason's mirror held up Nature's light;
Shew'd erring Pride, whatever **is**, is right; …
Reason and Passion, answer one great aim:
That true Self-Love and Social are the same;
That Virtue **only** makes our bliss below;
And all our knowledge **is**, ourselves to know.

Alexander Pope
Essay on Man, 1733

12

Ethics for research on humans

IN THIS BOOK, I HAVE PLACED EMPHASIS on clinical ethics applied in clinical situations. For most people, this is where the crunch lies. The historical roots of health ethics come from such ancient sources as the Hippocratic corpus and oath, the writings of Avicenna and Spinoza in the middle ages, the books of Thomas Perceval (1803–1876) and the Code of Ethics of the American Medical Association, first expressed in 1847. These sources were largely based on such principles as beneficence (do good), non-malfeasance (do no harm), justice (be fair towards all) and virtue (be good).

While these concepts evolved over a long period of time, ethical concerns in the field of research over the past five or six decades have been driven more specifically by the need to protect the human subjects involved. Although 19th-century French researcher Claude Bernard enunciated principles for ethics in clinical research, and some countries (notably pre-World War II Germany, who, amazing as it now seems), had codes of conduct for human research, little attention was paid to them, and almost none was paid to the question of whether or not they were applied by researchers.

One of the first clinical research trials concerned the discovery of how fresh fruit could be beneficial in preventing scurvy in the Royal Navy of the 18th century (see pages 212–13). Captain James Lind was faced with 12 men suffering from serious cases of scurvy. He divided the men into six treatment groups: two men received a quart of cider each day; two men were given 25 drops of elixir vitriol three times daily; two men were given two spoonfuls of vinegar three times daily; two men were given a half pint of sea water each day; two men received two oranges and one lemon daily; and two men were given an electuary (a medicine composed of powders and other ingredients, mixed with sugar water or honey into a pasty mass suitable for oral administration) three times a day. After six days, the men who had received the fruit were well enough to care for the others. Unfortunately, it was at this point that they ran out of oranges and lemons.

The quaintness of this study makes it noteworthy, especially because it is the reason Englishmen came to be known as limeys. It is sad to relate that the therapeutic benefit of this research lay hidden for close to 50 years; their Lordships of the Admiralty ignored it until it was brought to their attention by another nobleman of significant naval rank who could not be as easily ignored as Captain James Lind.

Lind's study can be criticized on a number of grounds: there is no mention of consent or how the 12 sailors were randomized into the six treatment arms, but they all knew they were ill so one may assume consent; it is most irregular to have one of those who recovered look after the ailing sailors in the remaining groups; with a dramatic recovery of

---

CLINICAL TRIAL FOR SCURVY IN THE BRITISH NAVY, WITH SIX TREATMENT GROUPS

On the 20th of May 1747, I took twelve patients (with) the scurvy, on board the *[H.M.S.] Salisbury* at sea. Their cases were as similar as I could have them. They all in general had putrid gums, with the spots and lassitude, with weakness of the knees. They lay together in one place, being a proper apartment for the sick in the fore-hold; and had one diet common to all, viz.; water-gruel sweetened with sugar in the morning; fresh mutton-broth often times for dinner, at other times puddings, boiled biscuit with sugar, etc; and for supper, barley and raisins, rice and currants, sage and wine, or the like.

- Two of these were ordered each a quart of *cyder* a day.
- Two others took twenty-five [drops] of *elixir vitriol*, three times a-day, upon an empty stomach using a gargle strongly acidulated with it for their mouths.
- Two others took two spoonfuls of *vinegar* three times a-day, upon an empty stomach, having their gruel and their other food well acidulated with it, as also the gargle for their mouth.
- Two of the worst patients, with the tendons in the ham rigid [hamstring muscle group] (a symptom none of the rest had) were put under a course of *sea-water*. Of his they drank half a pint every day, and sometimes more or less as it operated, by way of gentle physic.

- Two others had each *two oranges and one lemon* given them every day. These they ate with greediness, at different times upon an empty stomach. They continued but six days under this course, having consumed the quantity that could be spared.
- The two remaining patients took an **electuary**, the size of a nutmeg three times a day, as recommended by an hospital surgeon, made of garlic, mustard-seed, rad. raphan., balsam of Peru, and gum myrrh; and using for common drink, barley water well acidulated with tamarinds....

The consequence was that the most sudden and visible good effects were perceived from the use of *oranges and lemons*; one of those who had taken them, being at the end of six days fit for duty. The spots were not indeed at that time quite off his body, nor his gums sound but, without any other medicine than the gargarism of elixir vitriol, he became quite healthy before we came into Plymouth, which was on the 16th of June. The other was the best recovery of any in his condition and, being now deemed pretty well, was appointed nurse to the rest of the sick.

Next to the oranges, I thought the *cyder* had the best effects. It was indeed not very sound, being inclinable to be sour. However, those who had taken it were in a fairer way of recovery than the others at the end of the fortnight, which was the length of time all these different courses were continued, except the oranges....

As to the *elixir of vitriol*, I observed that the mouths of those who had used it by way of gargarism were in a much cleaner and better condition than many of the rest, especially those who used the vinegar, but perceived otherwise no good effects from its internal use upon the other symptoms....

There was no remarkable alteration upon those who took the *electuary and tamarind decoction, the sea-water or vinegar*, upon comparing their condition at the end of the fortnight, with others who had taken nothing but a little lenitive electuary and cremor tartar at time in order to keep their belly open....

Conclusion: As I shall have occasion elsewhere to take notice of the effects of other medicines in this disease, I shall here only observe that the results of all my experiments was that oranges and lemons where the most effectual remedies for this distemper at sea.... I am apt to think oranges preferable to lemons though perhaps both given together will be found most serviceable.

James Lind
"Treatise on the Scurvy" Edinburgh, 1753[121]

Ethics for research on humans

both men in the same group, the study should have been immediately stopped, and that therapy made available to all other groups; and if there was not enough fresh fruit for all the others, the ship's surgeon ought to have pestered the captain to put into the nearest port for fresh fruit for the remaining sufferers. Nevertheless, it resulted in a remarkably clear research outcome and one that heralded the science of clinical trials.

Lind's dramatic success did not prompt the development of guidelines for doing research on humans. Not yet. Indeed, no such guidelines were developed until Claude Bernard (1813–1878), a renowned French physiologist, enunciated principles for animal experimentation.[122] As amazing as it is, the country that took most seriously the ethics of medical research in human subjects in the early part of the 20th century was Germany. Their guidelines (see pages 214–15), developed before Adolf Hitler's election in 1933, were superior to any in the West, including the France, U.K., the U.S. and Canada.

It is a cause for deep deliberation and soul-searching that the great German medical profession—which led the world in sensitivity toward the protection of research subjects—could be suborned and ultimately disgraced by their lack of an organized protest against the enormities the Nazi regime enacted against those with mental disability or congenital developmental disabilities; elderly people with degenerative diseases; and later, against the Jewish people of Europe. It is a warning to us all.

 CIRCULAR OF THE REICH'S MINISTER OF THE INTERIOR CONCERNING GUIDELINES FOR NEW THERAPY AND HUMAN EXPERIMENTATION, ISSUED BY THE COUNCIL-HEALTH-COUNCIL (REICHSGESUNDHEITSRAT) 28 FEBRUARY 1931.[123]

Final Draft of Guidelines for New Therapy and Human Experimentation

1. Medical science, if it is not to come to a standstill, cannot…dispense completely with Human Experimentation. The special rights to be granted to the physician under these new guidelines must be balanced by the special duty of the physician to be aware of the grave responsibility which he bears for the life.

2. The term New Therapy…defines therapeutic experimentation which serves the process of healing.

3. The term Human Experimentation means operations and…research purposes which are non-therapeutic; it includes the side-effects and

consequences which can not yet be adequately determined on the basis of available knowledge.

4. Any New Therapy must be in accord with the principles of medical ethics,...both in its design and in its realization.

5. A consideration...of possible harms must...stand in a suitable relationship to expected benefits.

6. New Therapy may only be applied if consent or proxy consent has been given in a clear and undebatable manner following earlier appropriate information.

7. Introduction of New Therapy in the treatment of children and minors requires especially careful examination.

8. Medical ethics rejects any exploitation of social or economic need in conducting New Therapy.

9. New Therapy using living micro-organisms requires heightened caution, especially in the case of live pathogens.

10. New Therapy may only be conducted by the chief physician himself or, at his specific request and with his full responsibility, by another physician.

11. A written report on any new therapy is required, containing information on therapy design, its justification...

12. Publication of results of New Therapy must respect the patient's dignity and the commandments of humanity.

13. In addition, the following [are] requirements for human experimentation:

    a. Without consent, non-therapeutic research is under no circumstances permissible.

    b. Any human experimentation which could as well be carried out in animal experimentation is not permissible.

    c. Experimentation with children or minors is impermissible if it endangers the child or minor in the slightest degree.

    d. Experimentation with dying persons conflicts with the principles of medical ethics and therefore is impermissible....[P]hysicians...will be guided by a strong sense of responsibility toward the patients entrusted to them and...will maintain a readiness responsibly to seek relief, improvement, protection or cure for the patient along new paths, when the accepted and actual state of medical science, according to their medical knowledge, no longer seems adequate.

    e. In academic teaching, every opportunity should be used to stress the special duties of a physician undertaking New Therapy or Human Experimentation....

Although the research by Nazi physicians was condemned at the Nuremberg Trials (1946–1948), the resulting *Nuremberg Code* did not have a significant impact on the way research was conducted and, in particular, on the way human subjects were treated in Western countries. This was of grave concern, because with the explosion of knowledge in medical sciences since 1945, clinical research trials have become a major professional undertaking. During the first few decades after World War II, most of this activity was academic and carried out by clinical researchers in major medical institutions (teaching hospitals) or, in the U.S., in the National Institutes of Health (NIH). It was largely publicly funded and grants were dependent on rigorous peer review. As already noted, the growth of the annual research budget of NIH has been truly phenomenal—increasing from US$1.5 billion in 1970 to US$21 billion in 2000—and exceeds the effort in other countries by a large margin. In Canada, with the demise of the Medical Research Council and birth of the Canadian Institutes for Health Research (CIHR), publicly funded research has increased from about $5 million in 1960 to about $500 million by 2000.

Despite this increase in public funding, a much greater proportion of clinical trial research is sponsored by the pharmaceutical industry, partly in association with public funding by federal (CIHR) or provincial agencies, but mainly from industry development funds. The researchers, too, are increasingly funded by the industry, either as salary or through funds made available for recruiting patients into drug trials—sometimes very substantial amounts.

With the change in research funding sources came a change in who was conducting the research. Rather than lying strictly in the purview of academia, researchers began coming from non-academic sources, in particular physicians in private practice. When a physician enrols his or her patients in such research, there is potential for confusion and sometimes a poorly recognized conflict of interest. On the one hand, the physician-researcher has to assume the role and responsibilities of the physician (for patients) and, on the other, the responsibilities of a principal investigator for research subjects. The "best interests" calculus of each is not always the same. For the physician, the "patient's best interests" are of paramount import, whereas the researcher is committed to seeking "generalizable knowledge." Juggling both of these factors can create an ongoing conflict of interest for the physician, as well as conflicts of financial interests.

The accompanying lists lay out the background for research ethics. The examples of unethical research listed on page 216 provide some of the more heinous examples of unethical research. This list is not in any way complete, but it does give some of the examples that awoke the Western world, especially North America, to the ethical hazards of research on humans.

Most of these examples concern experimentation on patients without disclosure of risk, or informed consent (see Chapter 3 for details).[132] The list on page 221 provides some of the codes, guidelines and policies that were developed to guide and regulate human research. In the U.S., some of these were legislated and are controlled through regulations. All research now requires an ethics review, which is done by Institutional Review Boards in the U.S. and Research Ethics Boards (REBs) in Canada. Ethics review committees must approve each research protocol and attention is paid to the process of informed consent and information sheets. Researchers are made fully aware of the difference between "seeking their patient's best interests"—the therapeutic relationship—and "seeking generalizable knowledge"—the investigator relationship.

Clearly, the latter has special ethical risks for individual research subjects concerning the adequacy of information and their comprehension of it, and therefore the validity of consent. It is also the responsibility of REBs to look into such aspects as the research question, methodology, subject population, method of subject recruitment, statistical analysis of data, coverage of additional costs incurred, and to plan for reporting results.

These guidelines establish that duty to the research subject is paramount and informed consent is critically important. They evolved as the sheer quantity of research increased at an unprecedented rate, as the ethical issues grew increasingly complex, as technological and scientific advances were made, and as the role of the researcher evolved. My own experience was no exception.

Personal involvement in research ethics

I have been involved as an investigator in clinical research since the 1950s. I have described, occasionally with some remorse, some of the many dilemmas that I have encountered in clinical research.

The first concerned the management of infection of the valves of the heart with organisms (subacute bacterial endocarditis) which, though sensitive to penicillin, required extraordinary high doses of the drug for many weeks to get the desired cure (see Chapter 1 for details). It was a very successful venture that gave me great satisfaction, even though my role was confined to simply caring for the patients.

My next experience was at the Royal Post-Graduate Medical School in Hammersmith, London, in 1953 (see Chapter 3 for details). I was shocked to realize that two research studies conducted on patients with chronic liver failure (cirrhosis) while I was doing my residency were later considered by Henry Beecher to have been unethical.[133,134] On reflection, I have concluded that we were still in the era where the outcome *for the many* was often weightier than possible risk of harm *to the few* (*utilitarian* efficiency for social good outweighed the *deontological* duty to the individual). We also presumed a trusting relationship between researcher and the patient, in which the researcher would always act in the patients' best interests.

We now know that this approach is simply not good enough. There was much professional hubris in all this. Beecher was absolutely right to bring it to the world's attention. The 22 examples he cites largely document research at well-established, prestigious medical academic institutions that enjoyed a good reputation. Indeed, some of the researchers earned prestigious awards for the very research projects that Beecher indicted, and many later rose to the highest echelons of the medical world.

At the Royal Victoria Hospital, exploratory research led to our use of the semi-isolated small intestinal wall to wash the nitrogen end-products out of the blood of patients with kidney failure (see Chapter 5 for details) and the use of cross-circulation between two patients, one dying of renal failure, the other from liver failure (also Chapter 5).

In 1964, one of the patients on dialysis developed a wide spectrum of antibodies in her blood, presumably against the foreign antigens present in the blood of her husband and of the numerous blood transfusions she had received, which we conjectured might be *beneficial* in graft enhancement (see Chapter 4 for details). We tested this theory by placing a skin graft from the patient onto the husband's arm. At that time, we did not know about hepatitis B and C viruses or how to distinguish good antibodies from bad. In this instance, the husband developed severe jaundice (hepatitis), but fortunately he recovered and the skin graft was rejected in the usual time. I do not remember submitting a protocol to anyone other than my colleagues, nor did I have to answer any questions about the ethical propriety of what we had done to him.

In Alberta, I was involved in three major clinical research projects: the anti-lymphocyte globulin (ALG) trial conducted with material provided by the Connaught Laboratories on contract from the Medical Research Council (see Chapter 6 for details); the long-term monitoring of patients' blood and lymphocytes against the preserved cells from the cadaver donor spleen so that we could plot rejection activity at successive time points (see Chapter 7 for details); and the Canadian Multi-Centre Trial of Cyclosporin (see Chapter 7 for details). Informed consent was not an ethical issue in any of these studies, partly because the subjects knew that traditional treatments were poor; they embraced the new approaches. However, the studies were ethically suspect because the investigator was often also the treating physician; the patient's best interests may have been in conflict with the search for generalizable knowledge.

Participation in research ethics review

My involvement in the reading and evaluating the ethical aspects of research started at the Department of Medicine at the University of Alberta in 1975. This was around the time that ethics review was mandated for all clinical research, although the manner in which this was done was left up to each local research entity to decide. I well remember the following type of conversation: "Hey, John, this grant application has to be in Ottawa in two days and Joe is flying there tomorrow. I have the Ethics Approval form here. You don't mind signing it, do you? I have three other signatures already. I could give you an hour or so to look through the grant. When you've signed it, give me a call and I will come and pick it up. Thanks, I really appreciate it!"

By 1980, the procedure had been tidied up a lot. It was decreed by the MRC that a faculty REB or committee was the best way to minimize conflicts of interest between the grant applicants and the ethics evaluation process. Departmental REBs disappeared.

In 1985–1986, I was chosen to be on the MRC committee working group that was to generate *Guidelines for the Ethical Conduct of Research on Human Subjects*, which was eventually published in 1987 (page 221, document 4). Our group was chaired by Bernard Dickens, a health law professor at the University of Toronto and someone I came to respect and hold in great affection. The group also included a retired pediatrician, a judge, a professor of social medicine, a gerontologist, three research administrators, and a journalist. Three of the group were from Quebec. We met in Ottawa, Toronto, Montreal and Calgary, and had some fascinating discussions. The whole process was educational and enriching in many ways. It was also very challenging.

One member of the working group, the journalist, could not believe that the REB was not also involved in monitoring research studies to see if the ethical undertakings of investigators were, in fact, carried out in the way that they had promised. Although the pharmaceutical industry monitors clinical trials assiduously, their interest is focused on the accuracy of records and close observance of protocol—the aspects that will be looked at by federal regulators when the company applies to license the new agent; they are not concerned with the investigators' ethics.

Today, research studies are still only minimally monitored in Canadian clinical research. Why, you might ask? Surely, this is the least one can do to protect the interests of the subjects in research? Yes, it is, and the reasons it is not yet done are twofold: first, no academic wants to be seen in the role of ethics police by his or her research colleagues; and second, funds available are insufficient to do it more than minimally. The fact remains that increasing monitoring is the next step in Canada's ongoing quest to protect research subjects.

Still, the MRC working group made progress in establishing *Guidelines for the Ethical Conduct of Research on Human Subjects*. The term Research

CODES, GUIDELINES AND POLICIES TO GUIDE AND REGULATE HUMAN RESEARCH

1. The *Nuremberg Code* <www.ushmm.org/research/doctors/ Nuremberg_Code.htm>)
2. The Declaration of Helsinki (1964, revised in 1989 and 2000) <www.wma.net/e/policy/b3.htm>
3. The Belmont Report: Ethical Principles and Guidelines for the Protection of Human Subjects of Research, National Commission for the Protection of Human Subjects of Biomedical and Behavioral Research (1979) <www.musc.edu/research/ori/irb/links.htm>
4. The *Medical Research Council (Canada) Guidelines for Research Involving Human Subjects*, Ottawa (1987)
5. Social Sciences and Humanities Research Council (Canada), Ethics in Human Experimentation, Ottawa (1978)
6. WHO *International Ethical guidelines for biomedical research* involving human subjects. Geneva Council for International Organizations of Medical Sciences (1993)
7. The *Good Clinical Practice Guidelines* of the International Conference on Harmonization (U.S., Japan, Europe) and adopted by Health Canada in 1996
8. Canada's *Tri-Council Policy Statement for Ethical Conduct* for Research Involving Humans (1998), now widely adopted by the Canadian Institutes of Health Research as well as the two other Canadian research funding councils: Social Science and Humanities Research Council, and National Science and Engineering Research Council. <http://pre.ethics.gc.ca/english/ policystatement/policystatement.cfm>

Ethics Board was introduced in these guidelines to complement the American version of similar bodies: Institute Research Board. However, the Canadian system has been kept at the level of "guidelines," whereas the U.S. went for legislation to regulate the research ethics process. The advantages of legislation are a clearer definition of committee composition, jurisdiction, accountability, legal liability and accreditation criteria. Guidelines, on the other hand, connote voluntary compliance and offer flexibility and adaptability, less bureaucracy and less legal liability. In my view, efforts should be made to keep Canadian regulations as guidelines, but there is a real need for some sort of accreditation and accountability. In the end, legislation may be necessary.

Research Ethics Boards

I served on the REB of the Faculty of Medicine at the University of Alberta for 12 years and found it to be a taxing, though valuable, experience. Each REB was composed of 12 to 15 people, and included specialists trained in ethics and health law, an administrator, a member of the general public and a nurse. During the monthly meetings, which typically lasted four to six hours, ten to 15 separate grant requests were reviewed. Before the meeting, each grant was assessed in detail by at least two members of the REB, who then led the discussion at the meeting—though all members were required to look over each grant in a less exhaustive way to see if there were aspects of ethical importance. This preparation took two or three evenings each month.

The scientific merit of the proposal is decided by the peer-review committee of the granting body, such as MRC, the Social Sciences and Humanities Research Council, or Canadian Institutes of Health Research (CIHR); for those who were not funded by a national public research agency, the local REB also had to make a scientific assessment (poorly conceived science is unethical).

Much time was spent examining the contents of the Information Sheets and Consent Forms that research subjects are asked to read, digest and "comprehend" before they can truly give "informed consent." Above all, it is important that each subject should know about any possible risk, in language that they can fully understand—not an easy undertaking when one considers the diversity of those who might participate in research.

The viewpoint of the person who was a member of the general public was always considered. The nursing outlook was often crucial to one's own understanding of a project and its possible ethical traps.

All this effort added administrative duty for busy professionals and faculty members, and they were asked to assume it *pro bono publico*. There were no payments for reviewing a 100-page industry-sponsored, multi-centred clinical trial protocol, though perhaps there should have been. In the future, there almost certainly will have to be, as the number of research trials ever increases.

My last effort in this field took place after retiring from the University of Alberta and moving to Ottawa in July 1998. The 1998 *Tri-Council Policy Statement* (page 221, document 8) is an innovation for research ethics in Canada. For the first time, the three federal funding councils (National Science and Engineering Council, Social Sciences and Humanities Research Council, and MRC) agreed on policies for the broad range of ethical issues arising from research on humans in Canada. One can hope that the effects of this new statement will permeate the whole research community, from social sciences to post-licensure marketing of drugs, with a level of uniform ethical intention and with appropriate ethical flexibility.

In late 1998 and early 1999, I accompanied the MRC director of ethics, Dr. Francis Rolleston, on a series of visits to Canadian universities with medical schools. He went to all 16, but I was only able to go to 11. It was a great insight into the clinical research operation in Canada, the trials and tribulations of overworked REBs, and the overlap and difficulties of trying to include the social sciences in medical policies. I am convinced that the joint councils approach is the right one, although my own personal view is that the protection of research subjects in Canada should devolve into the National Council for Ethics in Human Research (NCEHR).

This body should be given more money so that it can truly liaise, accredit, educate and nurture the REB system in Canada, echoing the development of the U.S. Office for Protection from Research Risk, which was rebranded in 2000 by the NIH (the funding agent) as the Office of Human Research Protections, a body now quite distinct from the NIH. In my view, the bodies responsible for judging which applications should be funded are not the most suitable for judging whether there are flaws in REB process. The NCEHR can also review research not funded by government research agencies and establish contact with those REBs. Indeed, it has appointed a task force to look into ways of accrediting REBs, a move that may prove to be very helpful.

Who monitors clinical research outside public institutions?

In the last decade or so, many clinical projects have been carried out in the community by physicians working directly with the pharmaceutical industry, independent of universities and health authorities. These include Phase 3 clinical efficacy trials (mostly randomized multi-centred controlled clinical trials) and Phase 4 trials (mainly multi-investigator studies designed to assess the wider application of new drugs after licensure by Health Canada). Their research protocols may not be rigorously reviewed for either science or ethics. The science question suits the manufacturer, but the research question is not necessarily the most ethically appropriate or important for the public. This industry research must, however, be reviewed to meet the *Good Clinical Practice Guidelines* of the International Conference on Harmonization (page 221, document 7), which industry must observe.

This is done to a large (and largely unknown) extent by *private* REBs. As mentioned previously, the pharmaceutical companies monitor how the protocol is carried out, but they are looking for rigorous observance of rules, not the rigorous application of ethics. Further, private REBs may be financed by industry, creating conflict between the best interests of industry and those of the research subjects. In addition, private REBs do not have ongoing control over investigators after project approval. The REBs of universities and other public bodies, on the other hand, have this sort of ongoing control, and can request it if necessary.

No one is now directly addressing this possible lapse in good research ethics in Canada, except the College of Physicians and Surgeons of Alberta. It insists that if Alberta physicians are involved in the research, the College has a duty—emanating from its responsibility to monitor professional standards—to review projects that do not fall in the purview of the universities' or public health authorities' REBs. Thus, there are no private REBs in Alberta.

The next step in protection of all research subjects is for all REBs to be accredited and this was, in fact, the main recommendation of an NCEHR task force on the subject, which reported in March 2002.

This all sounds very complicated. Is it all really necessary? I hope that those who have read the accounts of lapses in research ethics in this book will have formed the firm opinion that it is!

A wider perspective in human research: research in the developing world

The guidelines listed on page 221 have established that duty to the research subject is paramount, and that informed consent is always critically important. Unfortunately, it may be that we are about to slip back into a frame of reference embodied by the idea that "doctor knows best" with regard to research being done in the developing world. Great vigilance is required.

More recently, Western researchers have started to conduct studies in the developing world, giving rise to new dilemmas. Should the standards for research ethics, widely accepted in the Western world, apply with equal rigour to research conducted by the developed world in developing countries? Furthermore, is this research being done in these countries because it will benefit them? Or, is it being done because it is easier to get enrolment?

How should we regulate research that is done in the developing world, where trials are cheaper and standards less exacting but where treatment, based on those trials, will be offered—and profits gained—in the more profitable developed world? The fact is inescapable that even if a drug is shown to be effective for a common problem, people in developing countries usually cannot afford the drug.

Take the question of *placebo* groups. In the developed world, the control group cannot be placebo (an inert substance) if there is an established effective regimen. A new drug, or new combination, must be tested against the "known best available." For a new drug that may only show marginal benefit, industry prefers to test against a placebo because their results will appear more impressive and conclusive. Researchers from a developing country easily accept this lesser standard because they cannot afford the established drug anyway. After all, why should not half the subjects be treated with something that might work, even if the other half are getting no treatment. But is it ethically acceptable for researchers from the West to adhere to this lower standard, even if researchers from the developing country are quite happy about it? Most say that it is not.

The immenseness of these questions can be seen in the AIDS epidemic in sub-Saharan Africa and South Africa. An impassioned ethical debate is currently underway concerning amendments to the World Medical Association's ethics document, the Declaration of Helsinki. The amendment stems from a controversy surrounding maternal-fetal HIV transmission trials in developing African nations in the mid-1990s. A placebo was employed in the trials because it was considered that the research subjects would never have access to the expensive treatments then available. Many critics were outraged at what they considered an exploitation of vulnerable research populations and agitated vigorously to revise the Declaration. In 2000, the Declaration was amended to state, among other things, that after a study every research subject should be "assured of access to the best proven prophylactic, diagnostic and therapeutic methods identified by the study."[135] At this writing, critics, including researchers, pharmaceutical companies and the U.S. Department of Health and Human Services are arguing that this "claim is impractical and unjustified and, if implemented to the letter, would prevent much research in developing countries from taking place."[136] And so the debate heats up.

In addition to the ethical treatment of human subjects, there is also the question of the Western world's priorities in research. For most of the world, research on a vaccine to prevent AIDS should be a priority over expensive (and highly profitable) therapy for the disease. In fact, the research is focused on therapy, not vaccines, because treatment is always

The most profound danger to world peace in the coming years will stem not from the irrational acts of states or individuals but from the legitimate demands of the world's dispossessed.

Of these poor and disenfranchised, the majority live a marginal existence in equatorial climates. Global warming, not of their making but originating with the wealthy few, will affect their fragile ecologies most. Their situation will be desperate and manifestly unjust.

It cannot be expected, therefore, that in all cases they will be content to await the beneficence of the rich. If then we permit the devastating power of modern weaponry to spread through this combustible human landscape, we invite a conflagration that can engulf both rich and poor. The only hope for the future lies in co-operative international action, legitimized by democracy.

It is time to turn our backs on the unilateral search for security, in which we seek to shelter behind walls. Instead, we must persist in the quest for united action to counter both global warming and a weaponized world.

These twin goals will constitute vital components of stability as we move toward the wider degree of social justice that alone gives hope of peace.

Some of the needed legal instruments are already at hand, such as the Anti-Ballistic Missile Treaty, the Convention on Climate Change, the Strategic Arms Reduction Treaties and the Comprehensive Test Ban Treaty. As concerned citizens, we urge all governments to commit to these goals that constitute steps on the way to replacement of war by law.

To survive in the world we have transformed, we must learn to think in a new way. As never before, the future of each depends on the good of all.

The Signatories (See Appendix 3 for a list of the signatories.)

---

more profitable than prevention. Can this inequity be controlled through ethical codes and guidelines? It is a big question and it implies ethical problems of a frightening dimension for countries that cannot afford more than a few dollars per head per annum in health care, yet are spending a large percentage of their gross domestic product buying arms from the West so that they can resist or undertake aggression. My thoughts go to the letter signed by 100 Nobel Laureates in December 2001 in honour of the centenary of the Nobel Awards, warning that our security hangs on environmental and social reform (see above).[137]

Underlying these issues is a basic philosophical tension: should research always be dedicated first and foremost to the welfare and interests of the individual research subjects (i.e., *deontologically* based), or are there circumstances in which the individual research subjects' interests can be subsumed by the interest of the greater numbers of others who live in a given community or culture (i.e., *utilitarian* based)? This is an ethical trap.

The justification for much of the unethical research since 1945 has been—usually expressed tacitly—that risk can be imposed on some research subjects when the potential community benefit is sufficiently great. David Rothman[138] mentions that this attitude, which justified putting soldiers at risk during World War II, may have carried over in the early post-war period into the philosophy that justified risk-taking for research subjects; this was a time when the subject was expected to trust the researcher to ensure that the risks would not be more than minimal. Such philosophy has been rooted out by the Declaration of Helsinki and the Belmont Report, but may be creeping in again as researchers attempt to justify research in the developing world. Dr. Marcia Angell, a recent past-editor of the prestigious *New England Journal of Medicine*, refers to this aspect as a smattering of "ethical imperialism."[139,140]

The future of research in Canada

In 2000, new legislation established the CIHR, which replaced the MRC. This inspired concept came from the final president of MRC, Dr. Henry Friesen, himself a noted international researcher in endocrinology. He spearheaded the task force in 1997–1998 that came up with a new concept for health research in Canada: a virtual network of 13 research institutes in social and medical sciences. It encompasses the societal and cultural dimensions of four domains: basic biomedical science, applied clinical research, research in health services and systems, and research in the health of populations. The concept was developed with the support of the federal minister of health at the time, Allan Rock.

The 13 institutes, which cover all the special areas of the health sciences, are each committed to four active principles: peer review, ethics, knowledge management and business development. This concept provides a great opportunity for restructuring Canadian health research and integrating ethics into each institute. It may also give more independence and prominence to the NCEHR with its special responsibility for REBs. I was privileged in the summer of 1999 to serve on an advisory subcommittee in ethics for this grand venture. There are plans to improve ethical processes in medicine, but the outcome depends on the dedication of resources—both human and financial. It must succeed: the future of ethical treatment of human research subjects depends on it!

No man is an island, entire of itself; every man is a piece of the continent, a part of the main. If a clod be washed away by the sea, Europe is the less, as well as if a promontory were, as well as if a manor of thy friend's or of thine own were. Any man's death diminishes me, because I am involved in mankind; and therefore never send to know for whom the bell tolls; it tolls for thee.

John Donne (1572–1631)
Nunc lento sonitu dicunt, Morieris
(Devotions upon Emergent Occasions, no. 6. 1624)

13

Sharing between people:
Transplantation relationships

THE WHOLE FIELD OF ORGAN TRANSPLANTATION is permeated with ethical issues, as is aptly illustrated by my career-altering experience with a patient who tried to buy a kidney (see Chapter 10). This is but one example among the seemingly endless range of unresolved ethical issues, including the following:

Brain death issues

How can one be sure that death from cerebral causes, so-called brain death, is actual death?

Is the brain dead definition of death ethically acceptable, or a strategy to promote transplantation?

Take the instance of a pregnant woman who sustains a ruptured arterial aneurysm, whose brain ceases to function totally and irreversibly, yet life-support measures enable nutrition, digestive and excretory functions to continue and the fetus to mature. If relatives wish, life support can be terminated by "declaring death from cerebral," or life support can be continued until the fetus is viable. How should such a dilemma be resolved?

Certain cultures were reluctant to accept the concept of brain death. Japan did not accept it as valid until 1997, and Denmark resisted until 1990.[141]

Religious or cultural issues

Are there religious or culturally based reasons against the use of organs from a dead body?

There are indeed. For example, the Shinto religion considers the practice to be sacrilege, though the Japanese reluctance to use organs from the dead is also cultural.[142,143,144] Certain other societies—for example India—find cadaver transplantation unacceptable even though it may not be specifically against the tenants of Hinduism.

Deceased donors' wishes

If a person has signed a donor card, is consent also needed from the grieving family after that person's death? Should donor authorization legislation be implemented?

This dilemma arises frequently. Consider the following example. M.S. (initials have been changed), a 45-year-old man, sustained a very severe head injury in a motor vehicle accident and was declared brain dead at a neurosurgical unit about 12 hours later. He had a driver's license with clear evidence that he wished to donate all his organs for transplantation should he suffer sudden death. The family was in shock and seemed inconsolable. When asked about organ donation, and on being reminded that M.S. had signed his organ donation consent on his driver's licence, his wife said, "Good Lord, No! Surely he has suffered enough!" and burst into tears. Her son, aged 20, said he would do what he could to console his mother and asked for ten minutes with her. At the end of this time, he said, "It is no use; my mother can think of nothing apart from her grief and how we are going to get through all this. I'm sorry." The donor co-ordinator told this to a senior member of the transplant team, who said: "When I was told about the card, I got in touch with the coroner who said that he had no need to do an autopsy. We have to clear this sort of death with him. Because there was a signed donor card, he said we could go ahead with organ retrieval." Were the transplant team acting ethically in going ahead with organ retrieval?

In a society where everyone accepts the possibility—however remote—of one day needing an organ by transplantation to prolong life, is it valid to presume that a deceased person's organs are available, unless that person made a written prior exclusion ("presumed consent")?

A living person can designate the recipient of his or her organ, so why can a donor not designate recipient(s) of his or her organs after death (directed donation)? If society accedes to this idea, how should one respond if the "direction" shows racial discrimination against certain potential recipients?

Ethics issues in regard to the donor

How do transplant professionals (doctors, nurses and others) show respect to the dignity of a deceased person, when the body is being used to provide vital organs and tissues?

The removal of organs from a dead person for transplantation can be a coarsening experience. The body should be treated with dignity when it is being eviscerated (albeit carefully and delicately), and after long bones, bone marrow from the spine, and large strips of skin are removed, the body should be sewn up in preparation for burial. The only way to overcome this, it seems to me, is to require sensitivity pre-education with repeated reminders and periodic meetings with those who have benefited as recipients. Only in this way can the true meaning of what is going on be brought to bear on the situation to help the health professionals cope.

Ethical implications surrounding efforts to increase cadaver organ donation

Should one increase family willingness to donate the organs of a deceased person using methods other than appeals to their humanity and beneficence? For example,

- *by societal recognition of their generosity?*
- *by paying for funeral expenses?*
- *by an educational grant for bereaved children?*
- *by a simple cash payment?*
- *by paying fair market values for suitable organs?*

The question is slowly evolving in the U.S. Recently, the American Medical Association issued guidelines[145] for pilot studies using financial incentives to increase the supply of organs from the deceased. These are:

1. consultation and advice is sought from the population within which the pilot study is to take place;

2. objectives and strategies, as well as sound scientific design, measurable outcomes and set time frames, are clearly defined in written protocols that are publicly available and approved by appropriate oversight bodies, such as Institutional Review Boards;

3. incentives are of moderate value and at the lowest level that can be reasonably expected to increase organ donation;

4. payment for an organ from a living donor is not a part of any study;

5. financial incentives apply to cadaveric donation only, and must not lead to the purchase of organs from the deceased's family;

6. the distribution of organs for transplantation should continue to be governed by United Network for Organ Sharing (UNOS), based on ethically appropriate criteria related to medical need.

Issues of ownership, safety, and subsequent allocation of organs

Once organs are removed from a body after death, to whom do they "belong" while out of the body: the transplant team, the donor's family or the State?

The problem here is that, in law, there is no "ownership" of a deceased body. The executors and next-of-kin have the duty of body disposal when it is released, but they do not own it. Nor does the deceased person own it. The matter is complex and needs clarification in all Western jurisdictions.

Assuming that the transplant team has the delegated duty to dispose of transplantable organs, what principles are used to decide to whom they should be given? Should there be public supervision over the application of such principles?

Is this organ allocation decision-making flawed by nepotism (as a result of undue influence of physicians), the influence of the media, social and economic status, social worth, etc.?

Consider, for example, the case of Mickey Mantle, an American sports hero in baseball for over four decades, who made it into the Baseball Hall of Fame in 1974. Mantle's liver began to fail in 1995 after 43 years of abusing alcohol. He was diagnosed with end-stage liver disease. Later, the doctors discovered it was much worse than they thought: he had a growing tumour in the centre of his liver. Mantle was placed on the

UNOS waiting list, which prioritizes patients according to urgency. Mantle was placed on Status 2, which signifies patients who are hospitalized so they can be kept stable (Status 1 patients are in intensive care and are expected to die in about a week), and moved to the liver transplant program in Baylor Medical Center. On June 6, 1995, the hospital held a news conference to announce that Mantle needed an organ transplant. A day later, a donor was found, and even though Mantle was sixth in line, he received the organ. This sparked a great deal of criticism. Did Mantle get bumped up to the front of the list because he was a celebrity? The matter was investigated by UNOS, which found that there was nothing irregular in the assessment of priorities in this case. But it raises the sort of questions that occur frequently. Another ethical question is whether self-inflicted liver disease from alcohol abuse should be treated with transplants at all, or only after a period of proven sobriety.

People awaiting organs on transplant waiting lists
In Canada, do those on transplant waiting lists have a "right" to an organ?
In a publicly funded health care system such as Canada's, are governments and professional bodies acting negligently if they do not adequately strive to provide the needed resources (organs and tissues) for procedures that are established as insured, medically necessary treatments (i.e., no longer in research development)?
Probably the only answer is along these lines: It is not possible to satisfy all those in need of all insured services at all times, even though there is a wish to do so. Services can only be made available within a health service that is committed to fair distribution of benefits to all.

Issues surrounding living, genetically related donors of kidneys (and liver segments)
Are live related donors always free of coercion from other family members?
In 1964, a brother donated a kidney to his sibling, who ran into serious problems. After the kidney donation failed, the donor said to me: "I guess the family will be satisfied with me now, anyway."

Are there ethical flaws in the concept of kidney sharing between families, when incompatibilities prevent donation within both families, but not between them?
Suppose, for example, a person (donor 1) is willing to donate to his or her sibling (recipient 1), but their blood groups are incompatible (e.g., the donor has type A, and the recipient has type B). Meanwhile, another

donor (donor 2) is type B, but is not compatible with his or her type A sibling (recipient 2). In this situation, donor 1 could donate to the recipient 2, and *vice versa*. This is termed an "ethically balanced" Paired Kidney Exchange.

Ethically, it is more complicated if donor 3 is blood group AB (and can only give to another AB recipient). Should donor 3 be encouraged to give to the next AB person on the Deceased Donor Wait List (DDWL) if, by so doing his or her desired beneficiary, recipient 3 (who is, say, group O), gets the next Deceased Donor (DD)? Or, would such a practice of "unbalanced PKE" lead to other group O individuals on the DDWL becoming progressively disadvantaged? This complicated situation is due to the frequency of ABO blood groups in the population: 45%, group A: 40%, group B: 10%, and group AB: 5%.

With the improved results from cadaver kidneys, is it still ethically acceptable to use live related donors rather than expanding efforts to find organs from cadavers? Is it ethical for surgeons to operate on people who are perfectly healthy? What price primum non nocere?

This question is raised not only with genetically related family live donors, but with emotionally related live donors and undirected live donations, and with altruistically motivated donors who do not designate the recipient. There is still a risk of the live donor having a serious medical complication, early or later on.

Is the long-term risk of removing a liver segment known?

The risks have been very well reviewed in 2000 by J.F. Renz and R.W. Busuttil[146] and in 2001 by D.S. Seaman[147] for adult-to-adult, live-related liver transplants (LRLT). But more than one hepatic adult-to-adult donor has died in the post-operative period,[148] which caused the Mount Sinai Medical Center in New York City to put its adult-to-adult LRLT program on hold—despite previous experience at that centre. In 2001, this centre reported on 109 LRLTs from 139 potential ABO-compatible healthy donors, aged 18 to 60 years. The average donor stay in hospital was six days. All of these donors but one are alive and well, and there were few complications. In children, patient and graft survivals were 87.6 per cent and 81 per cent at one year, and 80.9 per cent and 78 per cent at five years. In adults, recipient patient and graft survival rates were 85.6 per cent and 77 per cent at one year.[149]

BEYOND THE HIPPOCRATIC OATH

Issues with unrelated living donors
SPOUSES
Are spousal donors truly uncoerced? In cultures where wives may be seen as belonging to their husbands, should it be assumed, a priori, that a wife who wishes to give her husband a kidney has likely been coerced? How should this be handled, ethically, for families from those cultures?

How does one judge spousal donation in common-law marriages?

ALTRUISTIC STRANGERS
Although altruistic strangers must be truly admired for their generosity and humanity, should one not always suspect ulterior motives, possibly financial?

ORGAN VENDORS IN A LIVE KIDNEY MARKET
Is the concept of "rewarded gifting" ethically valid, or is this, as I suspect, an oxymoron?[150]

Should a fair market value be available for those who genuinely feel they have the right to sell one of their paired organs, such as a kidney, in a controlled organ-vending market?

This is presently forbidden by law in all Western countries, but has recently been advocated by a noted bioethicist in the U.K. under the conditions of a single purchasing agent, termed a "monopsonic system," such as the U.K.'s National Health Service.[151] This fleshes out ideas put forward by others[152,153,154] and shows that the ethics in this area are evolving.[155]

The concept of indirect altruism: the altruistic use of money for indirect benefits—also known as "dependent altruism"
The concept of indirect altruism supposes that a donor *gives* his or her kidney to a pool of kidneys, controlled by an appropriate third party (e.g., an ethics committee, non-profit organ regulatory body) under legal assurance that, by so doing, the donor obtains for a loved one a "monetary good" which he/she could not otherwise afford. In other words, the donor does not receive money for his or her kidney, but does receive a benefit (e.g., lifesaving surgery) for a loved one. This process is carried out by third-party regulators who are responsible for deciding what an acceptable benefit for the donor's loved one would be, and then for financing that benefit, or "monetary good." The money for this benefit comes from the purchase of the kidney either by a government insured

health service, or by rich patients on dialysis who purchase it for the benefit of all in the pool, and not directly for themselves. The more kidneys in the pool, however, the more likely is it that one will be allocated to a purchaser in the normal course of allocation.

Would such a system involve an unethical use of the money from sold kidneys—both to the donor's loved one, in the case of "indirect altruism," or to an appropriately selected person from the kidney transplant waiting list in the case of a "monopsonic market purchase"?
The third party adjudicator system is the crucial here, but the job is not an easy one. Consider these two scenarios:

1. A person from Egypt wants to obtain treatment for his daughter who has acute leukemia, but he cannot afford it. He applies to the third-party adjudicator to accept his kidney on the understanding that the third party will then pay for his daughter's treatment and subsequent care with money obtained from its sale.
2. A man with no post-secondary education and only a modest income decides that he would give up a kidney in exchange for the third party paying for two years of Harvard Law School for his son, who has secured a place there.

Would each of these cases be judged ethically acceptable by the third party? This, of course, is the problem with indirect altruism. The concept is ethical, but the process of adjudication is very difficult. It raises the question of what defines altruism in our society.

Xenotransplantation
With xenotransplantation, or inter-species transplantation, there is a danger of generating totally new retroviruses that could then spread into society. Can recipient consent to xenografting be accepted when there is, in addition, a wide societal risk of new xenozoonoses?
It seems, for example, that the HIV/AIDS virus, and the virus causing SARS (severe acute respiratory syndrome) may have been initially passed to humans from animals—from an African monkey in the first example, and Chinese civet cats in the second.
How does one assess risk from a virus that does not yet exist?

How does one get consent from a society under such circumstances?

Will industry fund adequate non-human, inter-species xenotransplantation before say doing pig-human trials, bearing in mind that the cost of the former is just as much as the latter? Only the human trials would be cost-recoverable, with long-term profit potential.

Industry is already investing several billion dollars in gene-modified animals (pigs). Will governments be able to afford to offer such special animals in a publicly funded health care system?

How will equitable access be maintained if the early results are favourable?

What about animal care and animal rights in this field? Pigs will probably spend their entire lives in a germ-free environment.

In 2002, clinical trials of xenotransplantation in Canada were put on indefinite hold. This moratorium was obtained by consensus from a process of public consultation carried out by the Canadian Public Health Association.[156]

THE WHOLE SPECTRUM OF TRANSPLANTATION SCIENCE

Are there areas of transplantation science that should be prohibited on moral grounds?

One such area would be the brain. Such transplants raise questions of loss of individuality. There are parts of the brain that might be ethically transplantable, but not enough is known yet. It may be that forms of "generative" or "regenerative" medicine using stem cells will control developments in this area of neurobiology, but all this is mere speculation at present.

As is the case with most ethical issues, there are no easy answers. Physicians, philosophers, lawyers and the like continue to hold congresses and write books to help resolve some of these issues, and I am no exception. In 1988, shortly after my career change to health ethics, I co-organized with Dr. Calvin Stiller (of London, Ontario) and Dr. Tony Monaco (a transplant surgeon at Deaconess Hospital, Boston), the first international congress dedicated to these questions. This Ottawa Congress, "Ethics, Justice and Commerce in Transplantation: a Global View," was co-sponsored by Health and Welfare Canada and the Transplantation Society. It was judged to be a great success, but regrettably only attracted 350 participants whose collective registration fees were insufficient to cover the costs of the many speakers who were sponsored from all parts of the world, including Europe, South America,

India, Middle East, Singapore and Africa. The proceedings of this congress were published in full.[157]

The second congress on ethics issues in this field was staged in Munich, Germany, in 1990 by Dr. Walter Land, a transplant surgeon who had attended the Ottawa congress and decided there should be a European event. I helped plan the program, which had a more philosophical flavour than the one in Ottawa. This event, which was co-sponsored by the European Society of Organ Transplant and the European Dialysis and Transplant Association, was attended by about 500 people—still not a large number for a congress of this significance. Again, the proceedings of this congress were published in full.[158]

It is impossible to estimate how much progress is made through congresses of this nature, but that is true of nearly all conferences, congresses and conventions. They are events where topics may mature and where thinking is progressively shaped by discussion in both plenary and private sessions, and the net effect, though impossible to quantify, is surely beneficial. Essentially this is because they are qualitative events.

My third fling in the area was through a book, *Ethical problems in dialysis and transplantation*,[159] which Kluwer Academic Publications in Holland asked a nephrology colleague in Edmonton, Dr. Carl Kjellstrand, to write. He generously invited me to be co-author and we planned it and invited 14 contributors from countries including the U.S., U.K., China, Egypt, India, Japan and Czechoslovakia. This also was a great experience and personally educational. It also sold quite well, perhaps because of the favourable reviews from colleagues in the U.S.

Still, because nephrology is a relatively new field, so too are efforts to grapple with some of the ethical issues arising from it. This is further complicated by the continued growth in technology. I will attempt to further illuminate one of the more pressing issues.

The kidney marketing debate

One persistent area of ethical concern is the question of whether we should establish a market for human kidneys. Clearly this has the potential of solving a supply problem and of making a certain number of individuals relatively well off. Although no one knows what the going rate for a healthy human kidney would be in the West, I would guess it would range from $10,000 to $100,000.

I recently responded to a challenge[160] in the *American Journal of Kidney Disease* to my view that the selling of kidneys should continue to be universally condemned. The challenge came from several very proper sources, including the Ethics Committee of the Transplantation Society, previous articles by J. Radcliffe-Richards et al.[161,162] and J.S. Cameron and R. Hoffenberg,[163] who raised the possibility for renewed consideration and debate.

I shall explore here in some detail the arguments that support the point of view that marketing human kidneys is ethically wrong.

We allow the sale of sperm and blood and human ova in many countries in the West (specifically the U.S.), but not Canada. There is no strong societal move to impose a moral sanction against those sales. Why should the underlying principles that apply to *renewable* human tissues not also apply to kidneys? Is it simply because they are *non-renewable*? If so, why the big difference when we know (from 40 years experience) that removing one normal kidney from young healthy people has no effect on their life in the large majority of cases, and the surgery has a serious complication rate of only 0.3 per cent? The organ may be regarded as *redundant*.

Currently, most people's moral intuition holds that marketing of vital human organs is wrong and repugnant. But recent articles in the medical literature have challenged us to reconsider whether that moral intuition is engendered because it is an affront to our deeper moral principles, or because the issue generates moral confusion on our part. We are asked to rethink whether our determination to proscribe the sale of organs is truly just or fair to those who live in abject poverty, or merely ethical imperialism?[164,165] Further, if these arguments are found to be persuasive and sufficient, should we not be prepared to rethink our repugnance and give more room for personal autonomy in these matters?

In *resisting* these pleas for greater recognition of personal autonomy, the following arguments are relevant:

1. If vital human organs become market commodities, they become "thingified." A society that promotes such trade is compromising its attitude toward individual human dignity and respect. To avoid this compromise, it is justifiable to place a limit on others' autonomy by preventing the sale of human parts in an organ market.

2. Professionals involved in such commerce would bear full responsibility for its moral shortcomings. The professional commitment to *promote only the welfare of people who seek help* (each as a moral equal, worthy of dignity and respect) would be seriously compromised.

3. In the long run, the respect accorded to the medical profession in society would be seriously eroded. The profession, as a whole, would be demeaned in the eyes of those who deplore the diminished *deontological* commitment (*that all individuals have value beyond price*) by its adoption of a mainly *utilitarian* ethic (*maximizing the good for the largest number, if they can pay*). Participating doctors might, in effect, be seen as living off the avails of a human kidney market.

4. There is also the issue of coercion. Should society accept that individuals' poverty and desperation can be the basis for irreversible one-time-only self-sacrificial acts—provided those individuals claim to know the implications of what they are doing and the decision is free of coercion? If so, who judges when coercion is present or not? Some libertarians might argue that it is both arrogant and paternalistic to claim that those who live in abject poverty cannot make good decisions. Just as those in prison are deemed incapable of making good decisions about volunteering for clinical research, those who live in abject poverty may be deemed to be vulnerable to a point where their decision-making integrity is compromised when they are tempted to sell parts of their bodies for large sums of money. As P.A. Marshall et al. state: "Poverty is perhaps the most significant factor in making a person vulnerable to coercion...despite the ease with which certain scholars celebrate autonomy and disregard the potential for exploitation when financial rewards are offered for organs." And, "the possibility for coercion is real and very stringent efforts would have to be taken to ensure the choice is truly voluntary under any market approach."[166]

5. A free market for kidneys ignores the right of community opinion to insist on placing limits to personal autonomy *for reasons other than physical harm to others*. An attempt will be made later to lay out *morally legitimate limits to individual*

autonomy. Societies consist of people in mutually dependent relationships (howsoever modern urban life seems to obscure this fact).

6. Organ commerce is an affront those whose concept of "reverence for life" is rooted in transcendent values in which each human body has a sanctity, however hard it is to define it what that means. Renee Fox, in a recent essay, decries the "economically deterministic, utilitarian, profit-oriented, desacralized outlook on the human body and psyche" as a profanation.[167]

I believe these six reasons outweigh the argument for permitting the full exercise of the autonomy principle in the selling of vital human organs in most societies. In my view, the system for indirect altruism is an ethically acceptable way of using money to provide monetary good to others—if it is properly introduced into society and regulated responsibly.

I also believe that rich people have the right to buy whatever health care they need when the prevailing community and political ethic permits it. This would *not* be the case for medically necessary therapy in some Western countries, such as Canada, which have a single-payer insurance system (government) and guaranteed universal access for such services, regardless of ability to pay. But in other societies, such as those that H.T. Engelhardt calls "societies of moral strangers who do not share a content-full universal ethic,"[168] both parties (sellers and buyers) might have those rights. But for these correlative rights to be put into ethical context, the society *also* needs to expressly agree that:

- it, as a whole, can live with the risks (psychological and spiritual) to community solidarity, while serving the health benefits of a limited number of individuals; and
- medical and other health professions agree, despite the risks to professional integrity, to take ethical responsibility for the inequities of such organ commerce.

How do we sustain the ethical claim that the human body is sacrosanct and that its organs should not be commodified?
No one has come up with a purely *reasoned* explication of the claim that the human body is sacrosanct, but the concept is linked to an associated claim that all people are morally equal, and therefore deserve to be

treated with dignity and respect. These concepts are also linked to Schweitzer's concept of "reverence for life." As a constellation of concepts, they constitute the ethical basis of all relationships between people living in disparate societies around the world. Valuing our human relationships is, I maintain, a global *moral intuition.*[*]

We readily accept our underlying human instincts of self-consideration, self-preservation and self-advancement as valid. But we also know that we are social beings who depend on each other and all others in society. We convince ourselves that we need a mutually supporting society. This leads us to develop *prima facie* moral obligations towards them.

In so doing, we make what David Hume called the *"is"* to *"ought"* transition; we see our human situation as it is and we intuit and affirm that we ought therefore to respect the dignity of each other as moral equals because of this observation. The mental process responsible for this change from an *observation* to an *obligation* (i.e., from a *fact* to a *value*) is not logical reasoning. Rather, it is a process based on inner feelings or, better, the promptings of moral conscience or *moral intuition.*

There is no proof that moral intuitions are correct or binding, yet they seem to be of critical importance. They are not supportable by reason alone. From a basis of moral *intuitions*, or promptings of moral conscience, we then use *reasoning* to test the validity of our intuitions, and then to derive principles and rules to guide our actions. Intuitions, of course, are not infallible. People may intuit different meanings from, or values inherent in, different situations. And those who share intuitions do not necessarily use reason to reach the same obligations. *This constitutes the process of ethical dialogue and the resolving of those ethical dilemmas that occur when moral intuitions or principles clash.*

As a result of the basic belief in the dignity and integrity of other human bodies, we *proscribe* all sorts of actions, which moral intuition leads us to believe are harmful or degrading to ourselves or other people,

---

[*] In this discussion, I am not placing weight on moral intuitions grounded *only* in religious doctrine or divine revelation. In organ commerce, we are dealing with questions that cut across cultural, religious, economic and political boundaries. Therefore, I am committed to trying to base discussion on the claims and principles of ethics common to all races and creeds. Recently, there have been attempts to delineate a universal system for human ethics (see Engelhardt 1992 endnote and see Miller RB. Ethics of paid organ donation and the use of executed prisoners as donors: a dialectic with professors Cameron and Hoffenberg. *Kidney Int* 1999;55[2]:733–7). My stance should not be construed as discounting or denying validity to moral intuitions based on religious convictions—they are just not being used here.

or are detrimental to our society. I attempt to tease out the reasons for these proscriptions in a later discussion about the limitations of autonomy (see also Table 13.1).

In the present discussion, I will continue to use the concept of moral intuition, or prompting of moral conscience or commitment, to *prima facie* values, knowing that they elude absolute reasons for holding them. However, these intuitions and precepts are no more elusive than the utilitarian calculus of the *greatest good for the greatest number*!

Affront to our moral intuitions: the nature of repugnance

When our moral intuitions are affronted, we feel sadness, disgust, anger, fear or repugnance. Many of us are repulsed at the thought of people selling parts of their body for profit. But can we rely on repugnance to determine action or policy? There seem to be two forms of repugnance: a serious affront to one of our deeply-held moral intuitions, and some action or thought that is so unfamiliar that it confuses our moral compass and leaves us unsure of how to react.

In the first form, repugnance is deeply felt and we turn to our principles and rules of action to reason how best to defend our moral intuition of wrongness.

In the second, a practice causes repugnance, which we recognize as a level of moral confusion. We may find ways of reasoning so that what was initially repugnant becomes morally acceptable under specific circumstances. An example of this is how we view interference with a dead body.

In our culture, there has always been revulsion about interfering with a dead body. Many people, including medical professionals, reacted with horror and disgust when the cadaver kidney program began in 1963 at McGill University. With time, the beneficial outcomes changed attitudes; repugnance was overcome in three situations: the need to learn anatomy from dissection, the need to learn more about causes of death from medical autopsies, and the practice of taking vital organs out of dead bodies and putting them into other people. It has come to be seen not as a *desecration*, but as a sort of *consecration*, transformed by the altruistic nature of the gift involved and the benefit conferred. And that is how it is to this day in most parts of the world.

If there are some uses of the human body that are considered valid, how does one reason that it is not valid for people to do what they want

Table 13.1 The dimensions of autonomy.

Full autonomy	Limited autonomy	
1	**2**	**3**
unlimited autonomy	autonomy from causing physical harm to others	autonomy from involvement from others (e.g., third parties)
Dangerous activities and habits: • skydiving • bungee jumping • motor racing • drinking alcohol • smoking cigarettes	Traffic laws Firearms Smoking cigarettes Offences against property Offences against the body	Physician-assisted suicide Active euthanasia Selling cigarettes or alcohol to children Selling, promoting street drugs Living off the avails of prostitution
Now accepted by most, formerly unaccepted: • Equality between women and men • Equality among races • Prohibition of slavery • Women's control over unwanted sex • Control over sexuality & conception • Interracial marriages • Cohabitation of unmarried couples • Cohabitation of same-sex couples	• Equality of out-of-wedlock children • Body dissection, autopsies • Cadaver organs for transplantation ⬅	⬅
Application to the realm of human organ commerce		
Theoretical freedom to buy or sell body organs	Abjectly poor potential organ sellers should be protected from exploitation by the rich	Third-party professionals should not to partake in organ commerce, but pursue all avenues for altruistic donation

Limited autonomy

4	5
autonomy from psychological or spiritual harm to society (taboos)	**autonomy limited by obligations to preserve the common good and community values**
Racial discrimination	Paying taxes
Incest, marriage between siblings	Military service during war
Eating human flesh	Mandatory reporting (infectious diseases, child abuse, etc.)
Using dead bodies, except where legal	Preservation of the natural world
Slavery	Acceptance of universal individual human rights
Cruelty to animals	
Taking illicit street drugs	

Former autonomy limitations:
- Inequality between women and men
- Husbands owning wives
- Inferiority of some races
- Prohibition of interracial marriages
- Prohibition of cohabitation of unmarried couples
- Prohibition of cohabitation of same-sex couples
- No legal status for children born out of wedlock
- Acceptance of slavery
- Death penalty for many offences
- Using dead bodies—anatomy (pre-16th c), autopsy (pre-19th c), transplantation (pre-20th c)

Application to the realm of human organ commerce	
Community solidarity is enhanced by altruistic giving and harmed by commodification of the human body	Sale of human organs prohibited by moral intuition (or taboo) or repugnance; a crucial question is whether the time is coming when this prohibition should be seen as an encroachment on a person's autonomy

with their own bodies—which, in this context, prohibits them from selling one of their kidneys for profit. To justify this prohibition, we need to further examine *the dimensions of autonomy, its free expression and the restraints that can be exercised by a society* (see Table 13.1).

The various ways in which public and professional paternalism restrict personal autonomy in other spheres of our lives are summarized in Table 13.1. We are naturally in favour of having as much liberty and personal autonomy as possible (Table 13.1, column 1), unfettered by constraints apart from the risk of physical harm to others (Table 13.1, column 2). Thus, one is at liberty to pursue dangerous activities and habits and unhealthy lifestyles even though, if these lead to outright injury or disease, one will depend on societal resources for rescue and subsequent care.

There are four types of restraint imposed on our autonomous actions:

- *Limited autonomy from causing physical harm to others* (Table 13.1, column 2): These are restraints on activities that might (a) cause direct physical harm to others, even unintentionally (constraints imposed by laws controlling traffic or firearms); (b) expose others to bodily harm (torture, child molestation or mutilation, female circumcision, rape, murder, street drugs, yelling "fire" in public places); or (c) appropriate the personal property of others, either physically (theft) or intellectually (reputation, plagiarism).
- *Limited autonomy from involvement from others* (e.g., third parties) (Table 13.1, column 3): These are restraints on activities that, although permissible to do for oneself (e.g., suicide), may not be promoted with or for others (assisted suicide, euthanasia, encouraging others to become addicted to smoking or street drugs, living off the avails of others through prostitution). These are limitations that are imposed on us when we act as an intermediary or third party, either as a member of society or as a member of a specially-entrusted group within a society (such as physicians).
- *Limited autonomy from psychological or spiritual harm to society* (Table 13.1, column 4): These are restraints on activities that are an affront to moral or ethical norms and intuitions of our society because they are seen as causing risk to societal and

psychological values or causing spiritual harm. They are sometimes called taboos. They can be described as repugnant, and include such practices as racial and ethnic discrimination, sex discrimination, female circumcision, incest, pedophilia, bestiality, cannibalism, and cruelty to animals.

- *Limited autonomy by obligations to preserve the common good and community values* (Table 13.1, column 5): These are restraints on our personal autonomy as a result of our obligation to act for the common good of society and the preservation of community values—for example, paying taxes, serving in the military, or reporting gross antisocial actions (suspicion of child abuse) or risks to others (infectious diseases, or breaking confidentiality when a life is threatened). These obligations also include preserving the environment because of a commitment to ecological integrity. In general, our personal autonomy is constrained by having to obey the law, framed as it is on our moral values. We also have agreed for the past 50 years to the principle of universal individual human rights.

One can find the root of these limitations on autonomy in certain national or international agreements, as well as in the underlying principles of contemporary bioethics and moral theology. It is more than 50 years since the UN Universal Declaration of Human Rights[*] was agreed upon. The guiding principles in Canada were framed in 1982 in the Canadian Charter of Rights and Freedoms.[§]

It is notable that there are *moral intuitions that were once strongly held* by our Western society as taboos or general prohibitions, but *that are now no longer in that category* (Table 13.1, column 4). Western countries have largely relegated them to the area of freedom of action between people with full autonomy (Table 13.1, column 1) and the practices have become new moral obligations and matters for respect. This transfer list includes acceptance and recognition of racial intellectual and moral equality (outlined by Jared Diamond[169]); interracial and inter-religious marriage;

---

[*] Full text of the Universal Declaration of Human Rights, adopted and proclaimed by General Assembly resolution on 10 December 1948, is available at http://www.un.org/Overview/rights.html (accessed Feb 2004).

[§] Full text of the Canadian Charter of Rights and Freedoms is available at http://laws.justice.gc.ca/en/charter/ (accessed Feb 2004).

full equality and civil rights for all women; the homosexual lifestyle; the granting of full civic rights to the physically disabled or mentally challenged; the right to suicide; the granting of full legal status to those born "out of wedlock"; and freedom from the crime of blasphemy. Other societies are much less liberal in some of these areas.

In regard to the taboo against desecration of the human dead body, certain practices have been transferred to column 1—notably the study of anatomy, the study of disease by medical autopsy, and the restoration of life by means of deceased persons' organ donation—but other taboos remain. A taboo itself usually specifies things *we must not do* (i.e., prohibitions), in accordance with the customs of a society. But they may also express things *we must not fail to do* (i.e., the failure to perform). These can be categorized into classes, and then sub-classes. Some of the classes of taboos are *sexual* (e.g., types of sexual intercourse, or sexual practice, such as pedophilia), *social* (e.g., public nudity, acceptable behaviour in public places), *speech* (e.g., swearing, forms of address), *eating* (e.g., human flesh, certain animals), and the *wearing of clothes* (e.g., *hijabs* and other head coverings, trousers for women). There is almost no limit to the list of taboos in daily living. Selling bits of one's body is still one of them, but taboos can change over time.

We have loosened the definition of "mutilation surgery" to allow live organ transplantation when based on an altruistic donation by competent persons, but other prohibitions against surgery on healthy persons persist, except in the area of improvement of physical attributes through plastic surgery.

The question still remains: Why should the right to sell and organ be kept in column 4, and not transferred to column 1? The argument put forward here is that if organ commerce, proscribed because it falls in column 4, were transferred to column 1, it would *offend the principles of respect for oneself and for others that are crucial for the longer-term concepts of social solidarity and mutual respect of all*. To commodify the body, to allow organs to become products, would undermine those concepts. I believe that the recognition of autonomy-based rights—to do what one wants with one's body—does not outweigh the harm that would later occur to these social and community concepts, although I admit that this is based on moral intuition and cannot be proved by reasoning. Others quite legitimately believe that this taboo should now be dropped, provided that there are appropriate controls that prevent the victimization of the poor.

If, by accepting certain proscriptions or limitations to personal autonomy one is acting paternally, so be it. Table 13.1 tries to put the limits to personal autonomy into perspective. Only column 2 is composed of limitations to autonomy based on the risk of physical harm to others. Yet this is the category that often comes to mind when one thinks about limiting autonomy. Even if society decided to allow organ commerce (transfer it to column 1), the participation of health care professionals in such market practices could still be proscribed. For them, participating as third parties in organ commerce is a practice that is offensive to most people in society and many would contend that it offends the respect and dignity owed by health care professionals to society as a whole (column 3). Health care professionals are specially entrusted to act as third parties in the interest of the health and well-being of the whole society. Society holds them in trust, but that trust must be continually earned.

I am *in favour of* the personal right to suicide, but *against* legalization of physician participation in a patient's suicide, except under very clearly delineated (and therefore paternalistically defined) conditions. Active euthanasia is in the same class, especially when impaired decision-making capacity has not been formally recognized. Although I am not in favour of penalizing teenage women if, as mature minors, they decide to go into prostitution, I would proscribe anything or anyone who would promote or connive in that practice or profit from it, including child abuse and third-party pimps. Obviously, early abuse in the home is a contributing factor to prostitution and society is right to insist on obligations of disclosure by anyone who suspects it. Special proscriptions should also be imposed on those who actively induce children to buy cigarettes or street drugs.

These are all examples of being in favour of accepting another's right, as a competent person, to certain actions that do not harm others directly, while paternalistically resisting (therefore favouring the proscription of) participation and promotion of such actions by *third parties* because of the potential of these actions to cause harm to others or to the fabric of society and, in the longer term, diminishing social solidarity. Although some may perceive a theoretical right to sell off parts of themselves to others, directly or indirectly through third parties, I intuit that such practices are ethically wrong and may, therefore, legitimately be proscribed.

Concerning the selling of human tissues (e.g., blood, skin) that are renewable or can be regenerated, the same arguments hold, but with much less force. It is still preferable, in my view, to obtain such tissues on a voluntary basis and to pay for their processing and distribution from the public purse, rather than to buy them from commercial outfits, mainly abroad, as Canada currently does. But a whole new set of issues are raised when renewable tissues (e.g., sperm, ova) are used to generate new people. Not only are the commercial aspects ethically questionable, but the creation of people through *in vitro* fertilization would only be ethically acceptable if the subsequently generated person has a legally protected right to his or her genetic history later on. They do not yet have this.

Future ethical issues in transplantation: toti-potential and pluri-potential stem cells

The prestigious journal *Science* referred to the discovery of the embryonic stem cell as the discovery of the year in 1999. There are several varieties of stem cells. Toti-potential means that a cell can differentiate into any cell in the body, and therefore, given the right modifying factors, can potentially grow into any organ in the body. Pluri-potential is a similar early cell, but with a more limited capacity for differentiation into other cell types. The original isolation of embryonic stem cells came from the inner cell mass of the very early embryo, at what is called the blastocyst stage. If transplanted into the inner cell mass of the early embryo of a genetically different strain of the same species—or even another species—these embryonic stem cells would grow along with the cells of the new host and the descendants of these transplanted cells would become part of the functional cells in all the host's tissues as the embryo matures, creating a *chimera*. Thus, these cells demonstrate two properties: their toti-potentiality for differentiation, and their acceptance by the new host's immune system as it matures (i.e., they achieve specific immune tolerance).

From the ethics standpoint, the first problem lies in obtaining these cells from human embryos. The nature of the dilemma is obvious. The U.S. government has addressed this aspect through the National Bioethics Advisory Commission, which published a two-volume report with recommendations early in the fall of 1999[170] in response to a request from President Bill Clinton in November 1998. The issue surfaced again with the George W. Bush administration in 2001.

It is still very early in this research, but the likelihood is that these cells will be available from other sources (e.g., cells in umbilical vein blood drained from the placenta after birth). Permanent cell lines (immortalized cell lines) have already been developed, and the future of this research is very promising. Society will have to respond variously to the ethical dilemmas as they arise.

It is easy to imagine the enormous implications of these findings for the field of transplantation. Perhaps the most dramatic application will be in the field of neurology, with the regeneration of nerves in the spinal cord or brain. Regrowing areas of a crushed or ruptured spinal cord would be a wonderful development for those people who are confined to wheelchairs. It is also possible that this technology could be used to grow new heart muscle fibres after muscle death from heart attacks. All this is a couple of decades into the future, but regenerative and generative medicine may be the areas of greatest advance as the new genetic knowledge is used in new ways.

Just as genes propagate themselves in the gene pool by leaping from body to body via sperms or eggs, so memes propagate themselves in the meme pool by leaping from brain to brain via a process which in the broad sense can be called imitations. ...

For more than 3000 million years, DNA has been the only replicator worth talking about in the world. But it does not necessarily hold these monopoly rights for all time. Whenever conditions arise in which a new kind of replicator can make copies of itself, the new replicators will tend to take over, and start a new kind of evolution of their own. Once this new evolution begins, it will in no sense be subservient to the old. The old gene-selected evolution, by making brains, provided the "soup" in which the first memes arose. Once self-copying memes had arisen, their own much faster kind of evolution took off. ...

We, alone on earth, can rebel against the tyranny of the selfish [gene] replicators...."

Richard Dawkins, *The Selfish Gene*[171]

14

Our evolving values

I HAVE TRIED TO WEAVE NEW INSIGHTS into the traditional values that underlie health care and human relationships, but how do we know these values are correct? How do we know if we can rely on them? What is there about them that makes them "better" than the values they replace? Are there absolute values out there that are faithfully represented by new values in health care? Are these values anything more than new ways of looking at the same old problems?

The early chapters of this book recount my medical career experiences during a period of exponential growth in knowledge and the attendant ethical dilemmas; the later chapters dwell on the ethics and values that have arisen. Looking back over the years, I am led to conclude that the evolution of health ethics was a driving force in my career.

In this last chapter, I attempt the difficult task of evaluating our values. Such an evaluation necessarily begins by examining how human ethics and values have arisen in the wider context of human evolution. I will contrast the concepts of evolution of gene characteristics (genetic evolution) with the evolution of ideas (memetic evolution) using the term "meme" to mean concepts or ideas. The opening quotation of this chapter indicates that I will apply, to a considerable extent, the ideas of Richard Dawkins, the Darwinian evolutionist who holds the Charles Simonyi Chair of Public Understanding of Science in that ancient seat of learning with its "dreaming spires," Oxford University.* (Although not subscribing to his atheism, I

---

* Richard Dawkins has written and edited a prominent series of books on the subject of Darwinian evolution, including *The Extended Phenotype*; *The Blind Watchmaker*; *River out of Eden*; *Climbing Mount Improbable*; and *Unweaving the Rainbow: Science, Delusion and the Appetite for Wonder*.

find his ideas inspiring.) I am also influenced by the writings of Dan Dennett[172] and Susan Blackmore[173]—both of whom have thought deeply about the concepts of memetics—and, more recently, Robert Aunger.[174]

Some elements of Darwinian evolution

The crucial replicating element of all biology is DNA as expressed through genes. The DNA molecule is several billion years old and has been making copies of itself all this time. In animals, the theory of evolution—through gene mutation and natural selection—dictates that changes in DNA structure, the enzymes and proteins they code, and then function, all start as mutations in the generation of an individual ovum or sperm. If its effect is beneficial to the survival of offspring, the mutated gene will gradually spread through the species, passing on the increased "fitness to survive" to the rest of the gene pool—survival of the fittest. This does not necessarily mean the fittest in any *physical* sense, but in a *reproductive or survival* sense. If environmental change dictates that fruit grow higher off the ground, this does not induce animals to have longer necks; however, if a random genetic mutation in ovum or sperm gives rise, quite by chance, to an offspring with a longer neck, that individual might have increased survival potential, and the mutation might then spread through the gene pool of the original species until a new species evolves. Those with longer necks will have been naturally selected genetically.

Evolution in species that are less evolved than humans (with the possible exception of some higher primates) is carried out entirely through genes. Nature—or survival pressure—does the selection. These species cannot consciously affect the selection process—it is governed by genes. This means that non-genetic factors for increased survival that an individual non-human animal may acquire during its lifetime (learning a new trick to obtain food or stumbling on a new way to escape from danger) are not reflected in its offspring's DNA and do not improve the survival of subsequent generations. There is no gene-independent transmission of culture or ways of doing things in the non-primate world.

Humans are different, in that they have consciousness and their ideas are passed on to their own as well as subsequent generations by non-genetic means—even through such memetic devices as the written page.

Genes and memes: nature and nurture

In the genetic sense, the human race evolves undetectably slowly. By comparison, human culture and society (knowledge, the arts and the incredible discoveries of science) are evolving with increasing speed. To address human cultural evolution, Dawkins coined the term "memetic evolution" (through memes) as a contrast to genetic evolution. To Dawkins, *memes* are cultural units that develop in the brains and minds of people in societies, which are then passed on or copied from brain to brain in a given generation, and, if widely approved, to subsequent generations by non-genetic replication. Our genes control the development of our brains (which have increased from a skull volume of 400 mL to 1500 mL over three million years of hominid evolution), but our ideas (memes), expressed through language and writing, have now taken control over how we live. Thus, religious world views are a collection of memes with increasing sophistication—meme-complexes—that describe visions of God. These visions have evolved in different parts of the world, and have succeeded in being passed on to successive generations.[*] Other cultural packages—memes or meme-complexes—include the works of Shakespeare, the music of Beethoven, computer science, the idea of professional sport, the mafia, the Beatles, jazz, gay and lesbian rights, and the development of ethics. Later in this chapter, I will develop the very concept of *health ethics* as a meme.

Those who read this book are exposing themselves to possible infection with new memes—even with the very concept of meme. Memes can spread through a population like an epidemic, except that they do not contain any DNA: think Jihad; think theory of Darwinian evolution; think Harry Potter.

Our *genes* enable us to think—they control the development of cognitive processes of the brain—but *memes* are the ideas and ideals that we think about.

---

[*] At this point, I am not going to get into the "ultimate truth" of "transcendental values" that deal with religious concepts and matters of personal faith. Suffice to say that I have been a practising Anglican all my life, albeit with strong reservations on certain quite important tenets of the Christian meme-complex!

Gender inequality in human societies

Take, for example, the issue of gender inequality in human societies. All agree that male control over females in human societies (demonstrated by females' lack of autonomy, treatment as property, lack of educational opportunity, sexual control through patriarchalism, economic dependency, etc.) is more prevalent than that observed in most non-human primate colonies. In some societies, women are still the property of their husbands—not to mention *purdah*, the *burqha*, the iniquitous dowry system for "selling" daughters, and the vicious perversity of female genital mutilation and female infanticide. So one must pose the question: Is gender inequality genetically or memetically determined?

This question provides an opportunity to discuss the dual roles of genetics and memetics in the development of human societies, and serves as a take-off point to discuss the relation between meme theory and ethics in general. Giant steps forward in the creation of cultures seem to have depended on two *non-human genetic* events:

1. the selective evolution of certain animals as a source of power for doing physical work. Wherever such working animals were indigenous, the emergence of farming cultures was favoured; and

2. the selective evolution of certain grasses and subsequent development of staple crops. The agrarian lifestyle enabled these people to prosper and multiply, and, above all, to have the time and leisure to develop ideas. From leisure came writing, and new ideas that led to politics, science and new knowledge—in a word, culture.

These two *genetic* processes (in certain animals and plants) were then consciously selected by humans who happened to inhabit those areas of the world. All this occurred during the last 13,000 years, and only in the parts of the world where these animals and plants were indigenous, but it enabled these human societies to replicate their memes.

As Pulitzer Prize winner Jared Diamond[175] adroitly points out: human cultures evolved differently, depending on where they were situated and which animals and plants they could control. Thus, the so-called superiority of European culture is a product of the fact that these Caucasoid races happened to originate in the fertile crescent of the Middle East. Similar explanations *favoured* human cultural emergence in China and *slowed* its emergence in the Americas, Australia and Africa.

It seems evident from study of human societies that the preferences and interests of human males have dominated in most human societies—though there have been some striking exceptions. But is this dominance *genetically* based, as in non-human primates, or is it primarily based on cultural concepts or ideas (i.e., on memes)? Clearly, the physical differences between men and women are determined genetically, but what about the conceptual differences?

Throughout most of history, and in most contemporary cultures, we see marked gender inequalities with male domination in such realms as politics, government, religion, policing and national defence,[*] and in the home. Male competitiveness (testosterone's effects) creates demands on males that may be expressed by increased aggressivity, and may underlie the fact that men commit most crimes, are responsible for most physical abuse and the vast majority of rapes, and populate prisons in a ratio of more than 10:1 over women. Male control over the levers of societal power, and thus educational opportunities, seem to have been responsible for male predominance in science, religion and public life (though in the realm of esthetics, the gender difference is minimal).

Since human male dominance over women seems to have been the norm throughout recorded history, does this mean that it must persist indefinitely into the future? Today, our answer, in the West, is no! New memes can now fight these old ones. That is the beauty of memes—they can resist any undesired behavioural properties that may reside in the old memes or in our *genes*. As Dawkins says, "We, alone on earth, can rebel against the tyranny of the selfish [gene] replicators."

In Western societies at least, the meme for gender equality is replacing the gender inequality memes that have been so widespread. We judge this to be a good thing—but that is an ethical statement!

---

[*] The evidence for nearly universal commitment to *militarism* is one of the most pathetic. Douglas Roche (*A bargain for humanity*. Edmonton: University of Alberta Press; 1993) describes the irony of $50 billion in arms being sold to Saddam Hussein by the West, who once viewed him as "a force of moderation in the Middle East." One reason for Iraq's invasion of Kuwait was to increase revenue to pay for these Western arms purchases. The 43-day Gulf war cost about $2 billion each day, although there was the opportunity to try out certain modern weaponry. The war was hardly over, he writes (p.26), "when the Bush (Sr.) administration announced a plan to sell five Middle East countries an $18 billion package of F-16 jet fighters, Patriot anti-missile defence, multiple-rocket launchers, and M-1 tanks." Even today, the largest budget item in developing countries in Africa is the purchase of military hardware.

What is the balance between genes and memes in ethics?

Ethics, though essentially a human enterprise, might have evolved first through genetic and then memetic stages. To justify this claim, we need to examine theories for the evolutionary origins of human behaviour in our primate ancestors.[*] I draw heavily at this point on views expressed by Australia's—now Princeton University's—philosopher ethicist, Peter Singer,[176] and such sociobiologists as Robert Axelrod[177] and Robert Trivers,[178] and John Maynard Smith and the philosophers Dan Dennett[179] and James Rachels,[180] who were all well reviewed by Matt Ridley in his 1998 book.[181,182,183,184,185] Their research traces the origins of behaviour in social animals and has identified several stages.[186,187] These include:

1. *Kin preference.* This encompasses behaviour to protect one's offspring, family and relatives in an extended family group. As we all recognize, the genes influencing caring for one's offspring are crucial for the survival of birds and mammals.

2. *Complex reciprocal behaviour.* This essentially incorporates the concept of you scratch my back, and I'll scratch yours. Among social animals, many biologists suppose that group members who lack genes for reciprocity may initially be at an advantage. For example, they may be better groomed, without the apparent need to do grooming in return. But in the long run, they will be at a survival disadvantage in such matters as mate selection. They would presumably be unaware of a sense of obligation (maybe I ought to have looked for skin ticks in the scalp of the chimp who picked out my skin ticks) or gratitude. Only if one supposes that non-compliant members are able to sense that they have done wrong, or feel guilty, does one enter the realm of ethics, the realm of norms and values, and the capacity to choose between them. There is no evidence that this is the case among non-human primates, though the matter is debatable—think of the behaviours of one's pet poodle!

---

[*] Strictly speaking, primates are our very distant cousins whose brains happen not to have evolved to the point of having comparable language skills based in abstract thinking (as far as we know), and they therefore have minimal memetic evolution.

3. *Apparent altruism.* This refers to co-operative animal behaviour that shows apparent willingness to act for the benefit of others, or a group of others, at the evident expense of one's own self-interest. This may be divisible into two categories: (1) where there is evident anticipated but *deferred self-interest*, and (2) where there seems to be *no* anticipated or consciously *deferred self-interest*. This second category is the most difficult to imagine because we understand so little about the ways higher social animals really think, or the extent to which they can conceive of abstract values and consciously choose among them. Some sociobiologists and many primate observers believe altruism occurs in non-human primates; other sociobiologists refute this, and interpret all apparent altruism as *occult selfishness* or *deferred self-interest* of some type.

When considering behaviour in non-primate mammals such as dogs, many observers (pet owners) attribute feelings of guilt and gratitude to them. Such speculation is not proof of an ethical ought/ought not system (comparable to human value systems). They can more readily be attributed to genetically programmed survival values, such as always behave towards the human who feeds you in ways that will be most likely to ensure your continued well-being and continued food supply—that is, your survival.

Behavioural biologists have a number of genetic models to explain co-operative behaviour. An example of co-operation activity, using the principle of deferred self-interest, is shown by wolves in fighting a cougar. The cougar could probably kill any number of lone wolves, but will succumb to a group of wolves who attack it as a pack (though perhaps killing one or two wolves in the process). In such situations, there are reasons to postulate *genetic* evolution of genes for co-operative action in wolves. Research is mute on whether they are free to choose *not* to act co-operatively.

Even such complex behaviours in social animals, which are not apparently motivated by self-interest (and which, therefore, might be construed as *altruism*), are not necessarily based on freely-made cognitive choices between values related *to survival of the other's genes* and those related to *one's own survival*. Only actions based on suppositions such as this could really be described as "ethical." They may be explained more readily as being gene-controlled strategies for indirect survival of the animal's own genes.

What it means to be ethical in *memetic* terms: Eth-memes

The challenge of ethics is to explain the transition from *is* (facts of nature or the natural properties of things) to *ought* (choice of action in accord with our norms or values with respect to good or bad, and right or wrong).

To act ethically, one needs to postulate:

> *First,* enough consciousness or cognitive development to have ideals and values, such as an ideal of altruism, gender equality, or the moral equality of all;
>
> *Second,* complete and unconditional freedom to choose among those values, using a norm for what is good or bad, and right or wrong; and
>
> *Third,* to be able to transmit our choices horizontally through a society, group or family, not just vertically from one generation to another.

For the present, we assume that although the higher social animals may act with *apparent* altruism in many situations, we are not able to establish that they consciously choose to act in this way because they think they *ought* to, or that they wish to affect the behaviour of other families or communities within that species.

Those who believe, from observing *animal* behaviours, that they can discern behaviours in response to *human* norms and values may be trapped in what G.E. Moore calls the "naturalist fallacy"[188]: trying to *define* human values in terms of the natural properties of things that illustrate those values. At the human level, we just know that we have concepts of values—altruism, beauty, virtue—even though we cannot *define* them by those natural properties that we appreciate through our senses (touch, smell, sight, sound and taste). *These values are just there as part of what we call consciousness.*

In the opinion of the behavioural sociobiologists, humans use their incredible cognitive capacity (carried to them through their genes) to develop value systems that are then expressed though memes and meme complexes. When acting to pursue their own self-interest, humans are frequently responding to influences of self-preservation through gene-driven behaviours. When acting against their own self-gratifying interests, they are more likely to be acting in response to meme-determined ideals or values. *Thus, meme-driven human behaviour sometimes conflicts with behaviour based on the evolutionary legacy of our genes.*

I will not explore the transition from gene-facilitated behaviour to meme-facilitated behaviour any further. Memes have been the most important units of cultural evolution since the beginning of human history. Indeed, one may claim that the narrative of human history, although revealing much behaviour that is gene-facilitated is, in fact, *the record of human meme evolution.*

In the rest of this chapter, the only memes considered will be those related to ethical behaviour. I have coined the term "eth-meme" to describe this category of meme, distinct from memes for music, warfare, religion and science.

Is there a problem in postulating that eth-memes drive the evolution of our culture so that we behave in ways that may conflict with behaviour that has gene-facilitated origins? Surely, the answer is: absolutely not. Our cognitive development has enabled us to modify and mould the natural world to conform to changing human ideas, both good and bad. Our inventiveness has given us material wealth, power, and improved health through science-based technologies. It has also given us the ability to exploit less advanced nations and affect our natural environment indiscriminately. Diamond claims that our hubris has led us to make unjustifiable claims to racial/ethnic genetic superiority.[189] Good or bad, by contemporary ethical norms, these culture-based factors are the products of memes acting largely independently of our genetic behavioural legacy.

As humans, we increasingly try to understand what is really meant by eth-meme ideals such as those embodied in the Golden Rule. I believe this concept is expressed by every religious system known to humanity, without exception. That notion is an evolving eth-meme. Thus, the global village eth-meme challenges the limits of more primitive genetic expressions of kinship and encourage us to make that particular transition from *is* to *ought. This, I contend, is the very nature of ethics.*

Hopefully, the word *eth-meme* has served the purpose of integrating the genetic aspect of behaviour with cultural evolution of behaviour, customs and traditions. Thus, to return to the initial question of gender equality, we can now iterate a new ethic, one that claims that moral equality between women and men means that women ought to be equal in every opportunity in life—especially in education, the workplace, and professional life—and ought to control all aspects of their lives and bodies in sexual and economic independence, with equality both in society and at home.*

Full adoption of the ethic of gender equality would bring this ethical dividend to a fuller understanding of the nature of all committed relationships that are grounded in mutual respect. Equality of this type would engender truly respectful relationships between people. It would also bring the justice and care perspectives of ethical practice into a *dynamic dialectic* that, perhaps, is *the essence of relational ethics.*

Does this establish our values and ethical principles as the right ones?

I have to say that it does not. There is no way of knowing, either by reasoning from principles or through moral intuition, whether our current values are absolute in any sense of that word. This does not mean that absolute truth and ultimate value and the universal love principle do not exist. We should anticipate that our values will evolve further in the future, just as we know they have evolved from the past. Indeed, we should welcome this moral uncertainty. As Kenneth Miller says in *Finding Darwin's God,*

> certainty of outcome means that control and predictability come at the price of [loss of] independence. By being always in control, the Creator would deny his creatures any real opportunity to know and worship him. Authentic love requires freedom, not manipulation. Such freedom is best supplied

---

* I will deal briefly here with the problem that the Judeo-Christian tradition has with regard to the notion of true gender equality. The inability of this tradition to deal adequately with this issue is a principal stumbling block to many people in the West. I contend that these religious traditions have serious conceptual (memetic) flaws in respect to such ideas as: God is the Father of Mankind; Christian revelation about the "humanity" of God has been framed in male imagery; only males, as priests in Christian Orthodox and Roman Catholic churches, can administer the sacraments; many churches support doctrines of women's dependency and inequality, in many facets of life, especially when married; and women are often not free to use new knowledge to control the natural processes of human reproduction. Such practices may be censured by the patriarchy.

I strongly affirm that Christianity accepts that there is moral equality in relationships between all men and women, even though, in practice, there is gender inequality, founded in certain flawed traditions. My ignorance of Islam prevents me from expressing a view on this matter there.

through the open contingency of evolution, and not by strings of direction attached to every living creature.[190]

The events described in this narrative have shown that our values in health care have been evolving and will continue to do so. I welcome, therefore, the open contingency of ethics, and hope that new knowledge of the nature of the world can be embraced more meaningfully in traditional meme complexes such as Christianity. Indeed, I find myself very attracted to the ideas of retired Episcopal Bishop John Shelby Spong of Newark, New Jersey, who has made himself a figure of controversy among his fellow bishops by thinking outside the box and accepting that we must embrace the notion of open contingency in Christianity.[191]

It is humbling to remember how much our values have changed. Did Christ unequivocally condemn slavery or gender inequality? No. Yet there is such beauty and grace in his life and his sayings (assuming that they are accurately recorded) that one can sense what he might teach on such 21st century issues as North/South disparity, global sales of military hardware and landmines, rampant tobacco marketing in the developing world, and environmental pollution. Think how the different influences of earlier puberty, greater educational opportunity, later marriages, knowledge of hormone cycles, development of anti-conceptional agents, and notions of gender equality have merged to change family values—to improve some of them, and to cause others to deteriorate—to suppose new ethical norms. This will continue in the future, perhaps at an ever increasing rate. Same-sex marriage is just another such issue.

What of health ethics in the future?

A final thought is to speculate on which of our current practices and values will develop further. I think about them in terms of *"levels of involvement,"* such as:

> *Level 1:* The individual's interaction with health professionals and their services.
>
> *Level 2:* Ethics issues at the community level and resource allocation of health services.
>
> *Level 3:* Ethics issues at a national level, especially the allocation of societal resources to achieve healthy lifestyles and prevent illness.

Level 4: Ethics issues in our global village that have an impact on health in general, within the concept of universal moral equality (e.g., healthcare in India). This includes man-made hazards (e.g., tobacco) and environmental aspects of health (e.g., climate change).

Level 5: Ethics issues such as advances in biological science that have an impact on the way we think about ourselves (our philosophies and faiths) and what we should or should not do, and how they change who we are and how we live.

It is not the function of this book to speculate on, or explore, all these ethical issues at their different levels. They are all part of the growing concept of memes. However, it is appropriate to develop some of the first-level issues, as every reader of this book will be involved with them in a personal way. The other levels will be left to evolve over time, and will include such questions as:

- When does a fertilized ovum become "ensouled" or merit being treated as a human being with legal rights, rather than merely a human life-form?
- Is it permissible to create new embryos to derive stem-cell lines for the purposes of therapy?
- Is there a role for reproductive cloning, if the reason is to help another person to live?
- Is it ethical to remove sperm from a previously consenting husband, recently deceased, so that a wife may conceive children through in vitro fertilization?
- What should be the obligations on those who live in affluence toward deprived impoverished people in other parts of the world?
- Through what political structures should the dictates of moral equality, as regards resources for health, be distributed to less advantaged people?

We, as a society, have already made significant inroads into considering the issues raised at first level of involvement: *the individual's interaction with health professionals and their services.* Consider, for example:

- *Consent.* There is little doubt in my mind that we must move from *informed consent* to *comprehended choice* by the patient, or a validly appointed patient surrogate. This may involve a new type of physician-patient relationship, requiring the involvement of other professionals—more or less along the model developed by the nephrology nurse clinicians (see Chapter 8)—so that patients will have a true understanding of their options before making their decisions. This understanding will come from someone who knows the patient, understands his or her values, and knows the patient's medical history. Such an advisor might play a crucial role in other aspects of patient care. This was formerly carried out by family physicians, who did it very well. Now, there is a shortage of such dedicated physicians and the role does not seem to attract doctors in the same way as it did in the past.

Nurses have developed the role of patient advocate, but I envision an expanded role that includes training in bioethics and research ethics, informed experience with end-of-life situations, and the ability to deal with the spiritual needs of patients in an advisory fashion. These advocates would become researchers and sources of information who are recognized by physicians, other health professionals and administrators, and would be given more status. Included in this expanded area of professional responsibilities are the consideration of advance directives and the appointment of surrogate decision-makers, especially with people over 65 years of age (though we should all give some forethought to such situations). The increasing complexity of health care seems to demand this.

Such individuals could be called "health care consultants"; their mandate would include familiarity with all forms of available treatment— public, public-private, private, or complementary medical approaches— and understand the implications of living in a multicultural society. These consultants would be available to everyone at public expense.

The word "patient" should be replaced by another word to indicate that those we currently label as patients are, in fact, vulnerable but fully participatory health care decision-makers. I do not know what term would be best—certainly not "client" or "user," as these two terms change the context of the relationship with health care professionals to one of the market place. This is fair enough for certain relationships (providing health protection, discussing events that carry no burden of vulnerability or risk), but are too impersonal for situations in which there is risk, pain or suffering. The best term may well be "person" or "individual with …" or some other "equality" terminology that still preserves the notion of human relationship.

- *Maintenance of human dignity.* One of the problems with the increasingly complex nature of health care is its tendency to become increasingly impersonal. For example, before a physician can determine the cause of an illness, many diagnostic procedures and professionals are involved, each providing an expert opinion. Of necessity, these professionals do not see the whole person, and it is almost impossible for them to think and act holistically. The factor that loses out is human dignity. We need to develop ethical strategies to counteract this tendency.

A very important component of ethical professional-patient inter-actions is establishing and maintaining *meaningful relationships*. This is also a key component of maintaining human dignity. The concept involved here is not only the relationship between professionals and patients, but also relationships between professionals. How does one maintain the concept that they are all involved with a person in need, not just fixing a complex multi-faceted system that is on the blink?

- *End-of-life situations.* There will undoubtedly be further developments in the way these situations are handled. One factor that drives physicians to undertake treatments— especially with older people—that are more extensive than they would probably accept or wish, is the fear of litigation. This area needs to evolve with new guidelines and new legal concepts. Physicians know that they are unlikely to be sued for doing the maximum to save a life, and that this defence is effective in justifying excessive end-of-life therapies. But is this right? Our society must continue to grapple with such questions.

  ○ Can people who are dying request assistance in bringing an end to their lives of suffering and deprivation? This is more active than merely being accorded the right to refuse treatment (which is now widely recognized as every competent person's right).

If physicians are to be enabled to provide such aid to the dying, new ways will have to be devised to involve third parties (including family members) and special legislation will be required to cover these special situations and afford appropriate protection to professionals.

- ○ In neonatal decision-making, the questions are more complex. How does one decide, using ethically defensible precepts, when life-sustaining efforts should not be pursued—even though it is technically possible—because that life might be considered to be too great a burden for the person and for all those responsible for that baby's welfare? Such decisions are fraught with all sorts of difficult questions.

- *The implications of a multicultural society.* Canada has become a society in which many cultures are treated with equality, both in society and at the individual level. The principle that we should adopt is one of respect and accommodation to these differences—provided that no harm is intended or comes to others. The value of these differences is evident at the personal level in such issues as the concept of individual autonomy (alien to some cultures, especially in the East) and, therefore, has implications for who is entrusted to make decisions at the family level. These values may also have an impact on who should deliver intimate health services, especially across genders. These different value systems need to be integrated into the way our society reflects different religious interpretations of life, especially in the level 5 type of issues.

I end this account of how we weave our values in health care with two quotations. The first combines hope in the future and implies confidence in what I hope may develop:

The [HIV/AIDS] epidemic continues its lethal march around the world, with few signs of slowing down. In the course of the past year, every minute of every day, some ten people were infected. In the hardest-hit regions, life expectancy is plummeting. [A]nd women now account for half of those infected worldwide....[T]he epidemic is expanding most rapidly in regions which had previously been largely spared—especially in Eastern Europe and across all of Asia, from the Urals to the Pacific Ocean....

But it is still my aspiration that health will finally be seen not as a blessing to be wished for, but as a human right to be fought for.

—*United Nations Secretary General Kofi Annan, 2003*[192]

My final quote was written by Prof. Solomon Benatar, a renowned health ethicist and physician in Cape Town, South Africa, and founder of its Centre of Medical Ethics. In his foreword to *Relational Ethics: The True Meaning of Respect*—a book which stems from the work of my colleague, Vangie Bergum and myself (largely her work, I must say)—he writes the following, which, I hope, describes how contemporary health ethics will develop in the future.

The scope and pattern of the bioethics endeavour has been considerably shaped by the notion that the world is made up of reflective, autonomous, self-determining individuals whose right to make choices for themselves is the most sacrosanct value in political life and health care. The value of community and of relationships had been undervalued and a dispassionate world of strangers constructed in which we are primarily responsible only for ourselves...a world in which money, power, bureaucratic processes, the law, technology and self-directed action increasingly dominate life.

There is a great danger of eroding the generosity, self-effacement, sharing, love compassion, empathy and solidarity required to link each of us to many others—within families, small communities, countries and the world. The capacity to imagine a better future is an integral aspect of macro-ethical relationships.[193]

It is my hope these thoughts become eth-memes for coming generations of health professionals and the politicians they elect.

Appendices

Appendix I

Advances in medicine over four epochs: 1760–2060

To fully appreciate the advances in medicine and the corresponding advances in medical ethics, I have divided modern medical history into four epochs: 1760 to 1880; 1880 until the start of World War II; 1940 to 2000; and 2000 to 2060, which is of necessity largely speculative.

The first (modern) epoch, circa 1760–1880

This was the age of clysters, cupping, nostrums and bloodletting. Many people did not survive into childhood and only a few, approximately 25 per cent, survived to old age.

The death of George Washington gives an interesting insight into the top medical people of the day (mid-December 1799). He was suffering from what would now be called a streptococcal throat infection with local abscess, or quinsy. For this he was treated with external blistering of the skin of the neck (surely the application of cantharides must have made things worse). He was orally administered a mixture of molasses, vinegar and butter. Another expert advised that he be given calomel (mercurous chloride) and tartar emetic (antimony potassium tartrate) and gargle with sage tea with vinegar. To top it all off, he was bled by a lancet into a vein on four separate occasions, to a total of 2,365 mL (80 fl. oz) of blood within a 12-hour period. His youngest physician, Dr. Elisha Dick, suggested performing a tracheostomy, which might have improved things, but the more senior consultants did not favour this. Small wonder that the first president of the United States expired![1,2]

The second epoch, 1880–1940

During the second epoch, the greatest improvement in health and longevity came from knowledge about the nature of infectious disease: controlling the spread of infection, antisepsis, improved sanitation, clean drinking water, vaccination and immunization.

Louis Pasteur (1822–1895) proved the nature of bacterial action when studying factors that made wine ferment (1840). This led to the formulation of the germ theory of disease, which Dr. Ignaz Semmelweiss (1818–1865), an obstetrician, applied to his practice from 1847 onwards. He showed that physicians who did not change their gowns or wash hands were responsible for the spread of infection from one obstetrical patient to another in hospital—the scourge of "puerperal sepsis"—though he did not publish until 1860. Then Joseph Lister (1827–1912) established the principles of asepsis for surgery in 1867. The scourges of humankind continued to be tuberculosis, puerperal fever, pneumococcal pneumonia (with a 25 per cent mortality rate; it is now 0.1 per cent among those in previous robust health), wound sepsis, and sporadic epidemics such as small pox. Indeed, World War II was the first war where more soldiers died from bullets than from disease.

Various childhood epidemic diseases took a vast toll, especially measles and diphtheria. Poliomyelitis was a scourge, but cancer, though it occurred of course, did not have the prominence in causing death that it has since attained. In 1909, the infant mortality rate for Montreal was 326 per 1000 live births (about one in three); in London, England, it was about one in four. It is now 5.2 per 1000, or about 0.5 per cent.[3]

This epoch presented a completely different medical world, as is evidenced by the changes in medical art. Paintings of physicians around 1900 typically depicted the physician sitting at the bedside of a sick child, perhaps dying of diphtheria, with a distraught mother nearby; a situation of empathy and powerlessness—accepting the inevitable with compassion. Thus, although the germ theory of disease had been established, there was precious little that could be done, apart from prevention.

But during this second epoch, there was great progress in the field of public health and preventive medicine. Indeed, these fields had first come into being during the previous epoch when Edward Jenner (1749–1823) showed, in a bold but very risky early experiment, that cow pox extract (a relatively mild pox disease of cows and dairy maids) could protect others from the much more virulent small pox—initiating vaccination

(1798) and other forms of protective immunology, such as active immunization. Jenner's experiment consisted of inoculating eight-year-old James Phipps with vaccinia (cow pox), waiting six weeks, then innoculating him with a fluid form of a variola (active small pox). He observed no infection, so the experiment was a success, but the ethics were dubious to say the least.

These preventive measures started the scientific assault against some of the common infections, which became an outright war, particularly during the second half of the 19th century. On the public health front, recognition of the value, and subsequent increasing use, of a pure sterile water supply and effective sewage disposal led to a great improvement in survival rates among the population, as reflected in increased longevity resulting from improved public health.

Although there were these great advances between 1880 and 1940, there were very few specific therapies for specific diseases, apart from insulin (1923) and thyroid extract. There was very little therapy available for non-infectious forms of disease. This period, however, was one where the diseases became increasingly well understood and the natural history of each described, even though little could be done to alter their course. It was a time for description of disease, and no one was more famous for this than Canada's Sir William Osler (McGill University, then Johns Hopkins in Philadelphia, and finally Regius Professor at Oxford University in U.K.). It was also a period of a great upsurge in the pathology of disease through autopsy of the dead—but not biopsy of the living, except for superficial lesions.

The third epoch, 1940–2000

Advances in the use of commonly known drugs are shown in Table A.1.

Two scientific discoveries of this recently completed epoch stand out above all others: understanding the structure of DNA and organ transplantation.

The structure of DNA was revealed to James Watson (1928–) and Francis Harry Compton Crick (1916–2004) in 1953,[4] when Watson was 25 years of age. From it came all our understanding of the way genes regulate the function of cells and body organs, and the wonderfully intricate ways in which cells turn on or off the generation of enzymes (with genes sending chemical RNA messages to ribosomes to make

Table A.1 A collection of agents now used in the management of assorted disorders, with discovery dates. It is by no means complete, but designed to provide a picture of the creativity of the third epoch.

Class of drug	Medication	Date	Principal effect	Significant scientist or science connection
Anesthetic	Ether	1842	unconsciousness in surgery; pain relief in obstetrics	W.T. Morton (Mass. General Hospital); James Simpson (Edinburgh), use in obstetrics
	Chloroform	1847		
Antibiotic	Sulphonamide	1933	early sulpha-drugs (Germany) shown to be non-toxic to humans; anti-TB—first controlled clinical trial of wide-spectrum antibiotics	Nobel 1939: Domagh for Prontosil, recd. in 1947; Nobel 1945: Florey, Chain, Fleming; Nobel 1952: Waksman, first semisynthetic antibiotic
	Penicillin	1941		
	Streptomycin	1948		
	Tetracyclines	1952		
Analgesics	Morphine	~300 BC	analgesia, cough/respiration; Peru/Bolivia coca-leaf analgesic; synthetic local anesthetic; local synthetic anesthetic	
	Cocaine	100s of years		
	Procaine	1905		
	Meperidine (Demerol)	1939		
Heart	Digitalis	~1775	slows racing heart; treatment for edema	1775, William Withering
	Mercurials	~16th C	acts at renal level—diuresis	Paracelsus, 16th c. (calomel) inhibits an enzyme (carbonic anhydrase) inhibits an enzyme (carbonic anhydrase) acts on nephron, not via carbonic anhydrase
	Acetazolamide	1930s	acts in kidneys—diuresis	
	Chlorothiazide	1957	acts in kidneys—diuresis	
	Ethacrynic acid	1963	acts in kidneys—diuresis	
Blood pressure diuretics	Beta-blockers	1969	blocks the sympathetic nerve; acts on cell receptors	
	Angiotensin CE-inhibitors	1975	dilates arteries; angiotensin formation is blocked	
Endocrine	Thyroid extract	1891	controls metabolism	1874 Myxedema; thyroid treatment from 1892; Nobel 1923: Banting/Best/Collip/McLeod; Noble 1952: Kendall/Hence/Recihstein; Structure—DuVignaud 1954, from posterior lobe of pituitary; Enovid—Pincus 1960, OrthoNovum: Butenandt isolates them in 1931
	Insulin	1921	diabetic control	
	Cortisone	1949	adrenal cortex deficiency	
	Anti-diuretic-hormone ADH	1953	controls diabetes insipidus	
	Estrogen	1930	feminizing agent in ovary	
	Progesterone	1962	control by estrogen/progesterone	
	Androgens	1932	masculinizing hormone	
Anemia	Ferrous salts	1831	Constituent of hemoglobin	Blaud's pills (1831), chlorosis (low iron) treatment; Nobel 1934: Minot/Murphy/Whipple
	Vitamin B12, folate	1948	from raw liver, cures P.A.;	
	Erythropoetin	1965	drives blood formation *in vivo*	

Class of drug	Medication	Date	Principal effect	Significant scientist or science connection
Vitamins	B1, B2, B6,B9	1926	necessary in diet; limes in sailor's diet eliminated scurvy; needed in diet, if lacking sunlight	Thiamine cures beri-beri; Nobel 1937: Szent-Gyorgi, vitamin C metabolism; cures, prevents rickets; produced by UV light to food or to the
	C	~1757		
	D	1924		
skin				
Tropical disease	quinine for malaria	~1650	controls fever, cinchona bark (Peru)	1935: kills *P. vivax* and *P. malariae* but not *P. falciparum*; 1941: Cowdrey—Dapsone for leprosy in rats and humans.
	anti-leprosy	1941	kills *Myco. leprae*, of Hansen, 1871	
Bubonic	antibiotics	1948	Streptomycin, tetracyline kills organism	see Antibiotics, above
Typhus	antibiotics	1948	Tetracycline, chloramphenicol kills Rickettsia	see Antibiotics, above
Cholera	antibiotics	1948	Co-trimoxazole & tetracycline kills *V. cholera*	see Antibiotics, above

certain proteins, using energy stored in mitochondria, and cellular debris being disposed of by lysosomes).

We can now listen to the chattering of cells in the body as they communicate their complex harmonics through hormones, cell receptors, interleukins (communicating molecules), integrins and the new techniques of genomics and proteinomics.

We are only just beginning to understand how genes work in teams to achieve even more complicated functions, such as the genetic control of behaviours or intelligence. It seems as if each week's new insight tells us more about the internal harmonies of the 30,000 or so genes in each cell of our body, and the sequence of letters in the billion or so words in the lexicon of life—the human genome. Research into the implications for human health is already under way. We have entered the age of applied molecular biology.

The fourth epoch, 2000–2060

Can we forecast what will influence longevity during our next epoch? Will the next leap forward come from applied genetics, new understandings of cell differentiation that allow us to grow new biopharmaceuticals (in "pharm-animals") and the ability to generate "spare parts" *in vitro* or *in vivo*, or will it stem from a fuller understanding of the influence on health and longevity of what we eat, what we inhale, what we think about and believe? Perhaps I can reveal my bias by citing two examples that point to the latter alternative.

First, there is the extraordinary research from D.J.P. Barker's unit for Environmental Epidemiolgy in Southhampton, U.K., that shows a significant difference in risk for coronary artery disease (CHD) in later life between two groups of men (all with comparable weight at birth of 3.5 kg [7.9 lb]). Children who weighed 8.2 kg (18 lb) or less at the end of the first year of life had a risk of CHD of 27 per cent, whereas those who weighed 11.8 kg (26 lb) or more at the end of the first year had a risk of nine per cent.[5,6] Similar results were obtained more recently in a study from Helsinki, which also showed an increased risk of CHD based on low birth weight. Thus, contemporary epidemiology research indicates that the way to prevent heart disease is through the better nutrition of young mothers during and after their pregnancies, so that they and their offspring are fully nourished, and through a good diet and exercise throughout life—not by planning for more open-heart surgical facilities.

Another example concerns the epidemic of obesity that is sweeping North America (and elsewhere), with its associated increasing incidence of type 2 diabetes (the common variety in adults), and that condition's complications of high blood pressure and chronic kidney failure. The incidence of kidney failure has doubled in the last 10 years, and the number of related deaths now exceeds the number of people who die from any form of cancer, except lung cancer; type 2 diabetes accounts for almost all of this increase.[7] The number one cause of type 2 diabetes is obesity (defined as being 20 per cent over ideal weight). In a study of 84,941 nurses over a 16-year period (1980–96), the relative risk (RR)— which gives the probability of diabetes in the higher risk groups compared with the probability of type 2 diabetes in the low risk group— is defined as 1.0 for those with a body mass index (BMI) of < 25.[8] For those with a BMI of 25–30, the relative risk was 7.6; for BMI 30–35, RR was 20.1; and for BMI of >35, the RR was 35. The other risk factors studied—lack of exercise, aspects of diet, smoking, and alcohol consumption—were much less significant.[9] Recently, a study from Finland has shown that the risk of type 2 diabetes can be lowered through diet and exercise. In this study, individuals at risk (with BMI of >30) were randomly assigned into two groups. Only one goup was intensively advised on weight reduction and exercise, and the incidence of the disease in this group was reduced over a four year period from 23 per cent to 11 per cent.[10]

Appendix 2

Some milestones in genetics[11]

SECOND EPOCH

1865 Abbé Gregor Mendel (1822–1844) publishes his studies on the inheritance of tallness, colour, and seed colour of strains of sweet peas from his monastery garden at Brunn. He demonstrated that trait heredity occurred as discrete units, which were independent of each other, and obeyed certain laws. His work was buried until 1902.

1902 Hugh DeVries, a botanist, rediscovered Mendel's work, and confirmed it with studies on the primrose.

1902 Archibald Garrod (1857–1936) shows that a human disease, alkaptonuria, is inherited in accordance with Mendelian laws.

1902 Walter Sutton (1877–1916) shows, in the grasshopper, that chromosomes carry inheritance factors. Recognizes the difference between phenotype (how it looks) and genotype (genetic makeup).

1905 William Bateson (1877–1916) suggests the new science should be called genetics—from the Greek genos, meaning birth.

1909 Wilhelm Johannsen (1857–1927), a Dutch botanist, suggests the word gene be used for the unit of heredity. J.H. Morgan begins definitive genetic studies with *Drosophila melanogaster*, the fruit fly. He was awarded Nobel Prize in 1933.

THIRD EPOCH

1941 George Beadle and Edward Tatum discover that genes act to regulate chemical reactions by enzymes. One gene, one enzyme theory.

1944 Barbara McClintock finds that genes can jump from one part of a chromosome to another.

1952 Hershey and Martha Chase discover that genes are made of DNA.

1953   James Watson and Francis Harry Compton Crick discover the structure of DNA, the unit of the genes, and trigger the new science of molecular biology.

1955   Arthur Kornberg discovers the enzyme DNA polymerase, opening the field of gene sequencing through use of the polymerase chain reaction of PCA.

1966   Marshall Nirenberg, Har Khorana, Severo Ochoa elucidate the genetic code—the codons (triplets) of bases that transport the 24 different amino-acids to RNA, which then builds them into proteins.

1983   First human disease gene (Huntingdon's disease) is mapped to chromosome four.

1990   Human Genome Project (HGP) is launched, together with the Ethical, Legal, and Social Implications of New Genetic Information (ELSI) project.[12]

1994   The US Food & Drug Administration approves the sale of the first genetically modified (GM) product, the FLAVR SAVR tomato.

1996   Mouse gene map completed.

1998   HGP map includes 30 000 genes.

1999   Mouse genome DNA sequencing completed; gene sequencing for human chromosome 22 also completed.

FOURTH EPOCH

2001   The DNA and gene sequences of the entire human genome are announced from two sources: one public, one private.

2002   The patent dispute over the cancer-prone Harvard onco-mouse reaches the Supreme Court of Canada. Scientists wish to patent the whole animal, not just the genes that make it cancer-prone.

Appendix 3

This letter was signed by 100 Nobel Laureates in December 2001 in honour of the centenary of the Nobel Awards, warning that our security hangs on environmental and social reform:

The most profound danger to world peace in the coming years will stem not from the irrational acts of states or individuals but from the legitimate demands of the world's dispossessed. Of these poor and disenfranchised, the majority live a marginal existence in equatorial climates. Global warming, not of their making but originating with the wealthy few, will affect their fragile ecologies most. Their situation will be desperate and manifestly unjust.

It cannot be expected, therefore, that in all cases they will be content to await the beneficence of the rich. If then we permit the devastating power of modern weaponry to spread through this combustible human landscape, we invite a conflagration that can engulf both rich and poor. The only hope for the future lies in co-operative international action, legitimized by democracy.

It is time to turn our backs on the unilateral search for security, in which we seek to shelter behind walls. Instead, we must persist in the quest for united action to counter both global warming and a weaponized world.

These twin goals will constitute vital components of stability as we move toward the wider degree of social justice that alone gives hope of peace.

Some of the needed legal instruments are already at hand, such as the Anti-Ballistic Missile Treaty, the Convention on Climate Change, the Strategic Arms Reduction Treaties and the Comprehensive Test Ban Treaty. As concerned citizens, we urge all governments to commit to these goals that constitute steps on the way to replacement of war by law.

To survive in the world we have transformed, we must learn to think in a new way. As never before, the future of each depends on the good of all.

The Signatories
(an asterisk appears beside the name of those
involved with medical ethical issues)

Zhohres I. Alferov Physics, 2000

Sidney Altman Chemistry, 1989

Philip W. Anderson Physics, 1977

Oscar Arias Sanchez Peace, 1987

J. Georg Bednorz Physics, 1987

Bishop Carlos Belo Peace, 1996

Baruj Benacerraf Physiol/Med, 1980*

Hans A. Bethe Physics, 1967

James W. Black, Physiol/Med, 1988*

Guenter Blobel Physiol/Med, 1999

Niclaas Bloembergen Physics, 1981

Norman E. Boriaug Peace, 1970

Paul D. Boyer Chemistry, 1997

Bertram Brockhouse Physic, 1994

Herbert C. Brown Chemistry, 1979

Georges Charpak Physics, 1992

Claude Tannoudji Physics, 1997

John W. Cornforth Chemistry, 1975

Francis H. Crick Physiol/Med, 1962*

James W. Cronin Physics, 1980

Paul J. Crutzen Chemistry, 1995

Robert F. Curl Chemistry, 1996

The Dalai Lama Peace, 1989*

Johann Deisenhofer Chemistry, 1988

Peter C. Doherty Physiol/Med, 1996

Manfred Eigen Chemistry, 1967

Richard R. Ernst Chemistry, 1991

Leo Esaki Physics, 1973

Edmond Fischer Physiol/Med, 1992

Val L. Fitch Physics, 1980

Dario Fo Literature, 1997

Robert Furchgott Physiol/Med, 1998

Walter Gilbert Chemistry, 1980

Sheldon L. Glashow Physics, 1979

Mikhail S. Gorbachev Peace, 1990*

Nadine Gordimer Literature, 1991

Paul Greengard Physiol/Med, 2000

Roger Guillemin Physiol/Med, 1977

Herbert A. Hauptman Chemistry, 1985

Dudley Herschbach Chemistry, 1986

Antony Hewish Physics, 1974

Roald Hoffman Chemistry, 1981

Gerardus 't Hooft Physics, 1999

David H. Hubel Physiol/Med, 1981

Robert Huber Chemistry, 1988

Francois Jacob Physiol/Med, 1975

Brian D. Josephson Physics, 1973

Jerome Karle Chemistry, 1985

Wolfgang Ketterle Physics, 2001

Gobind Khorana Physiol/Med, 1968*

Lawrence Klein Economics, 1980

Klaus von Klitzing Physics, 1985

Aaron Klug Chemistry, 1982

Walter Kohn Chemistry, 1998

Herbert Kroemer Physics, 2000

Harold Kroto Chemistry, 1996

Willis E. Lamb Physics, 1955

Leon M. Lederman Physics, 1988

Yuan T. Lee Chemistry, 1986

JeanMarie Lehn Chemistry, 1987

R.LeviMontalcini Phyl/Med, 1986

William Lipscomb Chemistry, 1976

Alan MacDiarmid Chemistry, 2000

Daniel McFadden Economics, 2000

César Milstein Physiol/Med, 1984*

Franco Modigliani Economics, 1985

Rudolf Moessbauer Physics, 1961

Mario J. Molina Chemistry, 1995

Ben R. Mottelson Physics, 1975

Ferid Murad Physiol/Med, 1998

Erwin Neher Physiol/Med, 1991

Marshall Nirenberg Phyl/Med, 1968*

Joseph E. Murray Physiol/Med, 1990*

Paul M. Nurse Physiol/Med, 2001

Max F. Perutz Chemistry, 1962*

William D. Phillips Physics, 1997

John C. Polanyi Chemistry, 1986*
Ilya Prigogine Chemistry, 1977
Burton Richter Physics, 1976
Heinrich Rohrer Physics, 1987
Joseph Rotblat Peace, 1995
Carlo Rubbia Physics, 1984
Bert Sakmann Physiol/Med, 1991
Fred. Sanger Chemistry, 1958; 1980
José Saramago Literature, 1998
J. Robert Schrieffer Physics, 1972
Melvin Schwartz Physics, 1988
K. Barry Sharpless Chemistry, 2001
Richard E. Smalley Chemistry, 1996
Jack Steinberger Physics, 1988

Joseph E. Stiglitz Economics, 2001
Horst L. Stormer Physics, 1998
Henry Taube Chemistry, 1983
Joseph H. Taylor Jr. Physics, 1993
Susumu Tonegawa Physiol/Med, 1997
Charles H. Townes Physics, 1964
Daniel T. Tsui Physics, 1998
Bishop Desmond Tutu Peace, 1984*
John Vane Physiol/Med, 1982
John E. Walker Chemistry, 1997
Eric F. Wieschaus Physiol/Med, 1982
Jody Williams Peace, 1997
Robert W. Wilson Physics, 1978
Ahmed H. Zewail Chemistry, 1999

Notes

1. Edelstein L, translator. *The Hippocratic Oath: text translation and interpretation.* Baltimore: Johns Hopkins Press; 1943.

2. Sass H-M. Reichsrundschreiben 1931: pre-Nuremberg German regulations concerning new therapy and human experimentation. *J Med Philosophy* 1983;8:99–111.

3. Wenzel RP, Edmond MB. Managing antibiotic resistance [editorial]. *N Engl J Med* 2000;343(26);1961–3.

4. Albert MR, Ostheimer KG, Breman JG. The last small pox epidemic in Boston and the vaccination controversy, 1901–1903. *N Engl J Med* 2001;344(5):375–9.

5. Alexander S. They decide who lives, who dies. *Life* 1962;53(Nov 9):102.

6. Scribner BH. Ethical problems of using artificial organs to sustain life. *Trans Am Soc Artif Intern Organs* 1964;10:209–12.

7. Levine DZ. Ethics Forum: Dossetor JB. On "Kidney vending: Yes! or No!" *Am J Kidney Dis* 2000; 35(5):1002–18.

8. Cates JE, Christie RV. Subacute bacterial endocarditis. A review of 442 patients treated in 14 centres appointed by the Penicillin Trials Committee of the Medical Research Council. *Q J Med* 1951;20(78):93–130.

9. Cates JE, Christie RV. Subacute bacterial endocarditis. A review of 442 patients treated in 14 centres appointed by the Penicillin Trials Committee of the Medical Research Council. *Q J Med* 1951;20(78):93–130.

10. Dossetor JB. Village practice on the Ganges Plain. *St Bartholomew's Hospital Journal* 1954;58(4):90 3.

11. Watson JD. *The double helix. A personal account of the discovery and the structure of DNA.* New York: Mentor/New American Library; 1968.

12. Lewin R. *In defense of the body: an introduction to the new immunology.* New York: Doubleday Anchor Original; 1974.

13. Jonsen AR. *The new medicine and the old ethics.* Cambridge (MA): Harvard University Press; 1990.

14. Beecher HK. Ethics and clinical research. *N Engl J Med* 1966;274:1354–60.

15. Rothman DJ. *Strangers at the bedside: A history of how law and bioethics transformed medical decision making.* New York: Basic Books; 1991.

16. White LP, Phear EA, Summerskill WHJ, Sherlock S. Ammonium tolerance in liver disease: observations based on catheretization of the hepatic veins. *J Clin Invest* 1955;34:158–68.

17. Welt LG. Reflections on the problems of human experimentation. *Connecticut Medicine* 1961;25:75–8.

18. Collins A. *In the sleep room: the story of the CIA in brainwashing experiments Canada.* Toronto: Key Porter Books; 1997.

19. Pappworth MH. *Human guinea pigs.* Boston: Beacon Press; 1967. p. 27.

20. Collins A. *In the sleep room: the story of the CIA in brainwashing experiments Canada.* Toronto: Key Porter Books; 1997. p. 244–5.

21. Collins A. *In the sleep room: the story of the CIA in brainwashing experiments Canada.* Toronto: Key Porter Books; 1997. p. 235.

22. Bickelmann AG, Burwell CS, Robin ED, Whaley RD. Extreme obesity associated with alveolar hypoventilaion: a Pickwickian syndrome. *Am J Med* 1956;21(5):811–8.

23. Merill JP, Murray JE, Harrison JH, Guild WR. Successful homotransplantation of human kidney between identical twins. *J Am Med Assoc* 1956;160(4):277–82.

24. Dossetor JB, MacKinnon KJ, Luke JC, Morgen RO, Beck JC. Renal transplantation between identical twins. *Lancet* 1960;2:572–7.

25. Dossetor JB, Morgen RO, Beck JC. Observations on the function of a transplanted kidney. *Can J Biochem Physiol* 1963;41:1409–22.

26. Scribner BH. Periodic hemodialysis for the rehabilitation of patients with terminal uremia. *J Clin Invest* 1962;41:1398–9, 1962.

27. Alexander S. They decide who lives, who dies. *Life* 1962;53(Nov 9):102.

28. Jonsen AR. *The new medicine and the old ethics.* Cambridge (MA): Harvard University Press; 1990.

29. Pateras VR, Dossetor JB, Gault MH, Helle SJ, Tagushi Y, MacKinnon KJ. The role of intestinal perfusion in the managements of chronic uremia. *Trans Am Soc Artif Intern Organs* 1964;10:292–7.

30. Taguchi Y, MacKinnon KJ, Helle S, Dossetor JB. A new method of intestinal perfusion for the management of chronic renal failure: a preliminary report. *Can Med Assoc J* 1963;89:252–4.

31. Kolff WJ. The beginning of the artificial kidney. *Artif Organs* 1993;17(5):293–9.

32. Gault MH, Rudwal TC, Engles WD, Dossetor JB. Syndrome associated with the abuse of analgesics. *Ann Intern Med* 1968;68(4):906–25.

33. Medawar PB. *The threat and the glory: reflections on science and scientists.* New York: Oxford University Press; 1991. p. 276–7.

34. Reemtsma K, McCracken BH, Schlegel JU, Pearl MA, Pearce CW, Dewitt CW, et al. Renal heterotransplantation in man. *Ann Surg* 1964;160:384–410.

35. Starzl TE, Marchioro TL, Peters GN, Kirkpatrick CH, Wilson WE, Porter KA, et al. Renal heterotransplantation from baboon to man: experience with 6 cases. *Transplantation* 1964;12:752–76.

36. Joyce LD, DeVries WC, Hastings WL, Olsen DB, Jarvik RK, Kolff WJ. Response of the human body to the first permanent implant of the Jarvik-7 Total Artificial Heart. *Trans Am Soc Artif Intern Organs*1983;29:81–7.

37. Calne RY, Alexandre JP, Murray JE. A study of the effect of drugs in prolonging survival of homologous renal transplants in dogs. *Ann N Y Acad Sci* 1962;99:743–61.

38. Murray JE, Merrill JP, Harrison JH, Wilson RE, Dammin GJ. Prolonged survival of human kidney homografts by immunosuppressive drug therapy. *N Engl J Med* 1963;268:1315–23.

39. Asamura H. The first transplant from a brain-dead patient in Japan. *Jpn J Clin Oncol* 1999;29(5):278.

40. Hekkinen JE, Rinne RI, Alahuta SM, Lumme JA, Koivisto ME, Kirkinen PP, et al. Life support for 10 weeks with successful fetal outcome after fatal maternal brain damage. *Br Med J (Clin Res Ed)* 1985;290(6477):1237–8.

41. Dossetor JB, Gault MH, Oliver JA, Inglis FG, MacKinnon KJ, MacLean LD. Cadaver renal homotransplants: initial experiences. *Can Med Assoc J* 1964;91:733–42.

42. Murray JE. Human kidney transplant conference. *Transplantation* 1963;2:149.

43. Editorial. *Ann Intern Med* 1964;60:311.

44. Starzl TE. Marchioro TL, Porter KA, Moore GA, Rifkind D, Waddell WR. Renal homotransplantation. Late function and complications. *Ann Intern Med* 1964;61:470–97.

45. Starzl TE. *The puzzle people: memoirs of a transplant surgeon.* Pittsburgh: University of Pittsburgh Press; 1992.

46. Dossetor JB, MacKinnon KJ, Gault MH, McLean LD. Cadaver kidney transplants. *Transplantation* 1967;5(4 Suppl):844–53.

47. Garg PP, Frick KD, Diener-West M, Powe NR. Effect of the ownership of dialysis facilities on patients' survival and referral for transplantation. *N Engl J Med* 1999;341(22):1653–60.

48. Kissmeyer-Nielsen F, Olsen S, Petersen VP, Fjeldborg O. Hyperacute rejection of kidney allografts associated with pre-existing humoral antibodies against donor cells. *Lancet* 1966;2(7465):662–5.

49. Taylor HE, Ackman CF, Horowitz I. Canadian clinical trial of antilymphocyte globulin in human cadaver renal transplantation. *Can Med Assoc J* 1976;115(12):1205–8.

50. Wilson, LG. The crime of saving lives. The FDA, John Najarian, and Minnesota ALG. *Arch Surg* 1995;130(10):1035–9.

51. Time for Najarian, U to go separate ways. *The Minnesota Daily* 1996 Feb 23 [editorial]. Available: http://www.mndaily.com/daily/1996/02/23/editorial_opinions/ (accessed February 2004).

52. Gault MH, Dossetor JD. *Nephron failure.* Springfield (IL): Charles C. Thomas Publisher Ltd.; 1971.

53. The reader may be interested in the rate of progress of genetics by considering the complexity of the HLA system. In the 1980s the two classes of HLA antigens (class I

and II) were being gradually worked out. Since then there has been a great expansion in the knowledge of the different alleles of each of these antigens, so that the number of known factors is almost 1,000. These dramatic changes can best be seen in the diagram below.

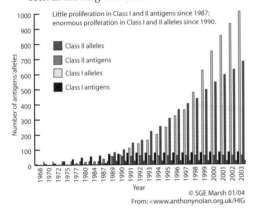

Little proliferation in Class I and II antigens since 1987; enormous prolferation in Class I and II alleles since 1990.

- Class II alleles
- Class II antigens
- Class I alleles
- Class I antigens

Year

© SGE Marsh 01/04
From: <www.anthonynolan.org.uk/HIG

54. Bach F, Amos DB. Hu-1: major histocompatibility locus in man. *Science* 1967;156(781):1506–8.

55. Bach FH, Albertini RJ, Amos DB, Ceppellini R, Mattiuz PL, Miggiano VC. Mixed leukocyte culture studies in families with known HL-A genotype. *Transplant Proc* 1969;1(1):339–41.

56. Dossetor JB, Howson WT, Schlaut J, McConnachie PR, Alton JDM, Lockwood B. *Study of the HLA system in two Canadian Eskimo populations. Histocompatibility testing.* Copenhagen: Munksgaard; 1972. p. 325–32.

57. Wachowich N. Sayiyuq: stories from the lives of three Inuit woman. *Globe and Mail* [Toronto] 2000 Feb 8; Sect R:1–2.

58. Morgan K, Holmes TM, Schlaut J, Marchuk L, Kovithavongs T, Pazderka F, et al. Genetic variability of HLA in the Dariusleut Hutterites. A comparative genetic analysis of the Hutterites, the Amish, and other selected Caucasian populations. *Am J Hum Genet* 1980;32(2):246–57.

59. Stiller CR, Dossetor JB, Carpenter CB, Myburgh JA. Immunologic monitoring of the transplant recipients. *Transplant Proc* 1977;9(1):1245–54.

60. Dossetor JB, Myburgh JA. Post-transplant immunologic monitoring: summation. *Transplant Proc* 1978;10(3):661–70.

61. Kovithavongs T, Schlaut J, Pazderka V, Lao V, Pazderka F, Bettcher KB, et al. Post-transplant immunologic monitoring with special consideration of technique and interpretation of LMC. *Transplant Proc* 1978;10(3):547–51.

62. The Canadian Multicentre Transplant Study Group. A randomized clinical trial of cyclosporine in cadaveric renal transplantation. *N Engl J Med* 1983;309(14):809–15.

63. Dossetor JB. Reminiscences of immunologic events in renal transplants: partial tolerance. *Transplant India* 2003;2(1):3–6.

64. Rajotte RV, Jirsch DW, Dossetor JB, Diener E, Voss WA. Survival of electrical activity of deep frozen fetal mouse hearts after microwave thawing. *Cryobiology* 1974;11(1):28–32.

65. Rajotte RV, Dossetor JB, Voss WA, Stiller CR. Preservation studies on canine kidneys recovered from the deep frozen state by microwave thawing. Proceedings of the IEEE. *Institute of Electrical and Electronics Engineers* 1974;62:76–85.

66. Grady D. Cell transplants offer hope for severe cases of diabetes. *New York Times* 2000 May 27;Sect A:1.

67. Shapiro AM, Lakey JR, Ryan EA, Korbutt GS, Toth E, Warnock GL, et al. Islet transplantation in seven patients with type 1 diabetes mellitus using a glucocorticosteroid-free immunosuppressive regimen. *N Engl J Med* 2000;343(4):230–8.

68. Flexner A. *Medical Education in the United States and Canada: A Report to the Carnegie Foundation for the Advancement of Teaching.* Washington (DC): Science & Health Publications, [1978?], c. 1910.

69. Rae A. Osler vindicated: the ghost of Flexner laid to rest. *CMAJ* 2001;164(13):1860–1.

70. Report vindicates Dr. Nancy Olivieri. *CAUT Bulletin Online* 2001;48(9). Available: http://www.caut.ca/english/bulletin/2001_nov/default.asp (accessed Feb 2004).

71. Robinson J. Nancy O. talks fast. In: *Prescription games: money, ego and power inside the global pharmaceutical industry.* Toronto: McClelland & Stewart; 2001. p. 115–35.

72. Robinson J. Taking aim at the doctors. In: *Prescription games: money, ego and power inside the global pharmaceutical industry.* Toronto: McClelland & Stewart; 2001. p. 193–215.

73. Eichenwald K, Kolata G. Drug trials hide conflicts for doctors. *New York Times* 1999 May 16; Sect 1:1.

74. Schweitzer A. *Out of my life and thought.* Baltimore: Johns Hopkins University Press;1998. p. 124–5.

75. Trivedi HL, Shah VR, Shar PR, Sane AS, Vanikar AV, Trivedi VB, et al. Megadose approach to DBMC infusion-induced allograft hyporesponsiveness in living-related allograft recipients. *Transplant Proc* 2001;33(1–2):71–6.

76. Bergum V, Dossetor JB. *Relational ethics: the true meaning of respect.* University Publishing Group For The Journal Of Clinical Ethics, Inc.; 2005.

77. Albrechtsen D, Leivestad T, Sodal G, Bentdal O, Berg KJ, Brekke I, et al. Kidney transplantation in patients older than 70 years of age. *Transplant Proc* 1995;27(1):986–8.

78. Dossetor JB. The selection of elderly patients for transplantation. In: Rosenthal RA, Zenilman ME, Katlic MR, editors. *Principles and practice of geriatric surgery.* New York: Springer-Verlag; 2000. p. 987–92.

79. Callahan D. Societal allocation of resources for patients with ESRD. In: Levinsky NG, editor. *Ethics and the kidney.* New York: Oxford University Press; 2001. p. 201–11.

80. Beauchamp TL. *Philosophical ethics: an introduction to moral philosophy.* New York: McGraw Hill College Div; 2001.

81. Beauchamp TL, Childress JF. *Principles of biomedical ethics*. New York: Oxford University Press; 1994.

82. Pellegrino ED, Thomasma DC. *A philosophical basis of medical practice: toward a philosophy and ethic of the healing professions*. New York: Oxford University Press; 1981.

83. Gilligan C. *In a different voice, psychological theory and women's development*. Harvard Univiversity Press, 1982.

84. Gilligan C. In a different voice. In: Singer P, editor. *Ethics*. New York: Oxford University Press; 1994. p. 51–6.

85. Engelhardt HT. *Foundations of bioethics*. New York: Oxford University Press; 1986.

86. MacIntyre A. *A short history of ethics: a history of moral philosophy from the Homeric age to the twentieth century*. New York: Macmillan Publishing Company; 1998.

87. Callahan D. *Setting limits: medical goals in an aging society*. New York: Simon & Schuster; 1987.

88. Jonsen AR, Toulmin S. *The abuse of casuistry: a history of moral reasoning*. Berkeley (CA): University of California Press, 1988.

89. Jonsen AR, Seigler M, Winslade W. *Clinical ethics: a practical approach to ethical decisions in clinical medicine*. New York: Macmillan Publishing Company; 1982.

90. Singer P. *Ethics*. New York: Oxford University Press; 1994.

91. Singer P. *Applied ethics*. New York: Oxford University Press; 1986.

92. Singer P. *The expanding circle: ethics and sociobiology*. New York: Oxford University Press; 1983.

93. Kuhse H, Singer P. *Should the baby live? The problem of handicapped infants*. New York: Oxford University Press; 1985.

94. Finnis J. *Natural law and natural rights*. New York: Oxford University Press; 1980.

95. Williams B. *Ethics and the limits of philosophy*. Cambridge (MA): Harvard University Press; 1986.

96. Reich WT. *Encyclopaedia of bioethics*. New York: Macmillan; 1987.

97. Rawls J. *A theory of justice*. Cambridge (MA): Harvard University Press; 1971.

98. Roy DJ, Williams JR, Dickens BM. *Bioethics in Canada*. Toronto: Prentice-Hall Canada Inc; 1994.

99. Bergum V, Schweitzer A, Dossetor JB, editors. *Ethics in the new age*. Vol 1. Edmonton: John Dossetor Health Ethics Centre; 1992.

100. Dossetor JB, Forbes D, Lambert T, Leraand GG, Ritchie C, Godkin D, editors. *Ethics in the new age*. Vol 2. Edmonton: John Dossetor Health Ethics Centre; 1999.

101. Dossetor JB, editor. *A handbook of health ethics*. Edmonton: John Dossetor Health Ethics Centre; 1997.

102. Ad hoc Committee to examine the Definition of Death, Harvard Medical School. A definition of irreversible coma. *JAMA* 1968;205(6):337–40.

103. Duff R, Campbell A. Moral & ethical dilemmas in the special-care nursery. *N Engl J Med* 1973;289(17): 890–4.

104. Jonsen AR. Critical issues in newborn intensive care: a conference report and policy proposal. *Pediatrics* 1975;55(6):756–68.

105. Optimum care for hopelessly ill patients. A report of the Clinical Care Committee of the Massachusetts General Hospital. *N Engl J Med* 1976;295(7):362–4.

106. Fried C. Terminating life support: out of the closet [editorial]. *N Engl J Med* 1976;295(7):390–1.

107. Bok S. Personal decisions for care at the end of life. *N Engl J Med* 1976;295(7):367–9.

108. Relman AS. The Saikewicz decision: judges as physicians. *N Engl J Med* 1978;298(9):508–9.

109. Steinbrook R, Lo B. Artificial feeding—solid ground, not a slippery slope. *N Engl J Med* 1988;318(5):286–90.

110. Angell M. Prisoners of technology—the case of Nancy Cruzan. *N Engl J Med* 1990;322(17):1226–8.

111. Dickens BM. Medically assisted death: Nancy B. *v.* Hotel-Dieu de Quebec. *McGill Law J* 1993;38:1053–70.

112. Sue Rodriguez *v.* British Columbia (Attorney General) (1993) 3 SCR 519.

113. Mendelson D Jost TS. A comparative study of the law of palliative care and end-of-life treatment. *J Law Med Ethics* 2003;31(1):130–43.

114. Beauchamp TL, Childress JF. *Principles of biomedical ethics.* 5th ed. New York: Oxford University Press; 2001.

115. Bernat JL, Mogielnicki RP, Gert B. Patient refusal of hudration and nutrition. An alternative to physician-assisted suicide or voluntary active euthanasia. *Arch Intern Med* 1993;153(24):2723–8.

116. Duff R. "Close-up" versus "distant" ethics: deciding the care of infants with poor prognosis. *Semin Perinatol* 1987;11(3):244–53.

117. Gillick MR. Rethinking the role of tube feeding in patients with advanced dementia. *N Engl J Med* 2000;342(3):206–10.

118. *Of life and death. Report of the Special Senate Committee on Euthanasia and Assisted Suicide.* Ottawa: Senate of Canada; 1995. Available: http://www.parl.gc.ca/english/senate/com-e/euth-e/rep-e/lad-tc-e.htm#m (accessed Feb 2004).

119. Lavery JV, Dickens BM, Boyle JM, Singer PA. Bioethics for clinicians: 11. Euthanasia and assisted suicide. *CMAJ* 1997;156(10):1405–8.

120. Stanley JM. The Appleton Consensus: suggested international guidelines for decisions to forego medical treatment. *J Med Ethics* 1989;15(3):129–36.

121. Brown SR. *Scurvy: how a surgeon, a mariner and a gentleman solved the greatest medical mystery of the age of sail.* Toronto: Thomas Allen Publishers; 2003.

122. LaFollette H, Shanks N. Animal experimentation: the legacy of Claude Bernard. *International Studies in the Philosophy of Science* 1994;8(3):195–210.

123. Sass HM. Reichsrundschreiben 1931: Pre-Nuremburg German regulations 124. Nuremberg Trials (1946–7). Facts on File News Services. Available: http://www.facts.com/icof/nurem.htm (accessed Feb 2004).

124. See http://en.wikipedia/wiki/NUREMBURG_trials.

125. Rothman DJ. Were Tuskagee and Willowbrook "studies in nature"? *Hastings Cent Rep* 1982;12(2):5–7.

126. Chamovitz R, Catanzaro FJ, Stetson CA, Rammelkamp CH. Prevention of rheumatic fever by treatment of previous streptococcal infections. I. Evaluation of benzathine penicillin G. *N Engl J Med* 1954;251(12):466–81.

127. White LP, Phear EA, Summerskill WHJ, Sherlock S. Ammonium tolerance in liver disease: observations based on catheretization of the hepatic veins. *J Clin Invest* 1955;34:158–68.

128. Krugman S, Ward R, Giles JP, Bodansky O, Jacobs AM. Infectious hepatitis: detection of virus during the incubation period and in clinically inapparent infection. *N Engl J Med* 1959;261:729–34.

129. Langer E. Human experimentation: cancer studies at Sloan-Kettering stir public debate on medical ethics. *Science* 1964;143: 551–3.

130. Collins A. *In the sleep room: the story of the CIA in brainwashing experiments Canada.* Toronto: Key Porter Books; 1997.

131. Cameron DE, Lohrenz JG, Handcock KA. The depatterning treatment of schizophrenia. *Compr Psychiatry* 1962;3:65–76.

132. Beecher HK. Ethics and clinical research. *N Engl J Med* 1966;274:1354–60.

133. Beecher HK. Consent in clinical experimentation: myth and reality. *JAMA* 1966;195(1):34–5.

134. Beecher HK. Ethics and clinical research. *N Engl J Med* 1966;274:1354–60.

135. Sibbald, B. Helsinki Declaration revisited over concerns about human subjects. *CMAJ* 2003;169(10):1066.

136. Sibbald, B. Helsinki Declaration revisited over concerns about human subjects. *CMAJ* 2003;169(10):1066.

137. Our best point the way. *Globe and Mail* [Toronto] 2001 Dec 7; Sect A:21.

138. Rothman DJ. *Strangers at the bedside: A history of how law and bioethics transformed medical decision making.* New York: Basic Books; 1991.

139. Angell M. Ethical imperialism? Ethics in international collaborative clinical research. *N Engl J Med* 1988; 319(16):1081–3.

140. Angell M. The Nazi hypothermia experiments and unethical research today. *N Engl J Med* 1990, 322(20):1462–4.

141. Program of the 2nd International Symposium on Brain Death. 1996 Feb 27–Mar 1; Havana, Cuba. Available: http://www.changesurfer.com/BD/1996/1996Program.html (accessed Feb 2004).

142. Morioka M. Bioethics and Japanese culture. Brain death, patients' rights, and cultural factors *Eubios J Asian Int Bioeth* 1995;5:87–90.

143. Religious faiths and transplantation. *TransPacific Renal News* 1997;April. Available: http://www.network17.org/pservices/relig.htm (accessed Feb 2004).

144. Kjellstrand CM, Dossetor JB, editors. *Ethical problems in dialysis and transplantation.* New York: Kluwer Academic Publishers; 1992.

145. American Medical Association. Cadaveric Organ Donation: Encouraging the Study of Motivation. Code of Medical Ethics E-2.151. Adopted June 2002. Available http://www.ama-assn.org/ama/pub/category/10827.html (accessed Feb 2004).

146. Renz JF, Busuttil RW. Adult-to-adult living donor liver transplantation: a critical analysis. *Semin Liver Dis* 2000;20(4):411–24.

147. Seaman DS. Adult living donor liver transplantation: current status. *J Clin Gastroenterol* 2001;33(2):97–106.

148. Gorman Christine. The ultimate sacrifice. *Time* magazine 2002; Jan 28:37.

149. Miller CM, Gondolesi GE, Florman S, Matsumoto C, Munoz L, Yoshizumi T, et al. One hundred nine living donor liver transplants in adults and children: a single-center experience. *Ann Surg* 2001;234(3):301–11.

150. Murray TH. Organ vendors, families and the gift of life. In: Youngner SJ, Fox RC, O'Connell LJ, editors. *Organ transplantation: meaning and realities.* Madison (WI): University of Wisconsin; 1996. p. 101–25.

151. Harris J, Erin C. An ethically defensible market in organs. *BMJ* 2002;325(7356):114–5.

152. Radcliffe-Richards J, Daar AS, Guttmann RD, Hoffenberg R, Kennedy I, Lock M, et al. The case for allowing kidney sales. *Lancet* 1998;351(9120):1950–2.

153. Friedlaender MM. The right to sell or buy a kidney: are we failing our patients? *Lancet* 2002;359 359(9310):971–3.

154. Rapoport J, Kagan A, Friedlaender MM. Legalizing the sale of kidneys for transplantation: suggested guidelines. *Isr Med Assoc J* 2002;4(12):1132–4.

155. Drukker A. Payment for organ donation: unacceptable or a possible solution? *Pediatr Nephrol* 2003;18(2):198–9.

156. Animal-to-human transplantation: should Canada proceed? A public consultation on xenotransplantation. Ottawa: Canadian Public Health Association; 2001. Available: http://www.xeno.cpha.ca/english/finalrep/reporte.pdf (accessed Feb 2004).

157. First International Congress on Ethics, Justice and Commerce in Transplantation: a global view. Ottawa, Canada, August 20–24, 1989. Proceedings. *Transplant Proc* 1990;22(3):891–1054.

158. Land W, Dossetor JB, editors. *Organ replacement therapy: ethics, justice, commerce.* New York: Springer-Verlag; 1991.

159. Kjellstrand CM, Dossetor JB, editors. *Ethical problems in dialysis and transplantation.* New York: Kluwer Academic Publishers; 1992.

160. Levine DZ. Ethics Forum: Dossetor JB on "Kidney vending: Yes! or No!" *Am J Kidney Dis* 2000;35(5):1002–18.

161. Radcliffe-Richards J, Daar AS, Guttmann RD, Hoffenberg R, Kennedy I, Lock M, et al. The case for allowing kidney sales. *Lancet* 1998;351(9120):1950–2.

162. Radcliffe-Richards J. Nephrarious goings on. Kidney sales and moral arguments. *J Med Philos* 1996;21(4):375–416.

163. Cameron JS, Hoffenberg R. The ethics of organ transplantation reconsidered: paid organ donation and the use of executed prisoners as donors. *Kidney Int* 1999;55(2):724–32.

164. Angell M. Ethical imperialism? Ethics in international collaborative clinical research. *N Engl J Med* 1988 319(16):1081–3.

165. Angell M. The Nazi hypothermia experiments and unethical research today. *N Engl J Med* 1990, 322(20):1462–4.

166. Marshall PA, Thomasma DC, Daar AS. Market human organs: the autonomy paradox. *Theor Med* 1996;17(1):1–18.

167. Murray TH. Organ vendors, families and the gift of life. In: Youngner SJ, Fox RC, O'Connell LJ, editors. *Organ transplantation: meaning and realities.* Madison (WI): University of Wisconsin; 1996. p. 252–72.

168. Engelhardt HT. The search for a universal system of ethics: post-modern disappointments and contemporary possibilities. In: Kjellstrand CM, Dossetor JB, editors. *Ethical problems in dialysis and transplantation.* New York: Kluwer Academic Publishers; 1992. p. 3–19.

169. Diamond J. *Guns, germs and steel: the fates of human societies.* New York: W. W. Norton; 1997.

170. Ethical issues in human stem cell research, September 1999. Rockville MD: National Bioethics Advisory Commission. Available: http://www.georgetown.edu/research/nrcbl/nbac/pubs.html (accessed Feb 2004).

171. Dawkins R. *The selfish gene.* New York: Oxford University Press; 1989.

172. Dennett DC. *Darwin's dangerous idea: evolution and the meanings of life.* New York: Touchstone; 1996.

173. Blackmore S. *The meme machine.* New York: Oxford University Press; 1999.

174. Robert Aunger. *The electric meme: a new theory on how we think.* New York: Free Press; 2002.

175. Diamond J. *Guns, germs and steel: the fates of human societies.* New York: W. W. Norton; 1997.

176. Singer P. *The expanding circle: ethics and sociobiology.* New York: Oxford University Press; 1983.

177. Axelrod R, Hamilton WD. The evolution of cooperation. *Science* 1981;211(4489):1390–6.

178. Trivers RL. The evolution of reciprocal altruism. *Q Rev Biol* 1971:46:35–57.

179. Dennett DC. *Darwin's dangerous idea: evolution and the meanings of life.* New York: Touchstone; 1996.

180. Rachels J. *Created from animals: the moral implications of Darwinism.* New York: Oxford University Press; 1991.

181. Ridley M. *The origins of virtue, human instincts and the evolution of cooperation.* Penguin Books; 1998.

182. Kitchener P. The evolution of human altruism. *J Philos* 1993;90:407–516.

183. Axelrod R. *The evolution of cooperation.* New York: Basic Books; 1984.

184. Trivers RL. The evolution of reciprocal altruism. *Q Rev Biol* 1971:46:35–57.

185. Sigmund, K. *Games of life: explorations in ecology, evolution, and behaviour*. Oxford: Oxford University Press; 1993.

186. Kriegman D, Knight C. Social evolution, psychoanalysis, and human nature. *Soc Policy* 1988;Fall:49–55. Available: http://www.comw.org/socbio899.html (accessed Feb 2004).

187. Nowak MA, Sigmund K. Cooperation versus competition. *Financial Analysts Journal* 2000;July–August:13–22. Available: http://www.aimr.com/pdf/perspectivesjaug00.pdf (accessed Feb 2004).

188. Moore GE. *Principia Ethica*. Cambridge: Cambridge University Press; 1903.

189. Diamond J. *Guns, germs and steel: the fates of human societies*. New York: W.W. Norton; 1997.

190. Miller KB. *Finding Darwin's God: a scientist's search for common ground between God and Evolution*. New York: HarperCollins Publishers; 1999.

191. Spong JS. *A new Christianity for a new world: why tradition faith is dying and how a new faith is being born*. San Fransisco: HarperSanFrancisco; 2002.

192. Kofi Annan. Message on World AIDS Day 2003 [press release]. Geneva: World Health Organization. Available: www.who.int/entity/hiv/events/wad2003/wad2003 (accessed Feb 2004).

193. Benatar SR. Foreword. In: Bergum V, Dossetor JB. *Relational ethics: the true meaning of respect*. University Publishing Group For The Journal Of Clinical Ethics, Inc.; 2004. In press.

Notes to Appendices

1. Morens DM. Death of a president. *N Engl J Med* 1999;341(24):1845–9.

2. Flexner JT. *Washington: the indispensable man*. New York: Mentor/New American Library; 1979. p. 400–6.

3. Wooltorton E. CMAJ, 90 years ago. *CMAJ* 2001;165(12):1631–4.

4. Watson JD. The double helix. *A personal account of the discovery and the structure of DNA*. New York: Mentor/New American Library; 1968.

5. Fall CH, Vijayakumar M, Barker DJ, Osmond C, Duggleby S. Weight in infancy and prevalence of coronary heart disease in adult life. *BMJ* 1995;310(6971):17–9.

6. Eriksson JG, Forsen T, Tuomilehto J, Osmond C, Barker DJ. Early growth and coronary heart disease in later life: longitudinal study. *BMJ* 2001;322(7292):949–53.

7. Hostetter TH. Prevention of end-stage renal disease due to type 2 diabetes. *N Engl J Med* 2001;345(12):910–2.

8. BMI is given by weight in kg divided by height in metres squared. A 100 kg (220 lb) person who is two metres tall would have a BMI of 100/4 or 25; someone who weighs 120 kg (264 lbs) and is the same height would have a BMI of 120/4 or 30.

9. Hu FB, Manson JE, Stampfer MJ, Colditz G, Liu S, Solomon CG, et al. Diet, lifestyle, and the risk of type 2 diabetes mellitus in women. *N Engl J Med* 2001;345(11):790–7.

10. Tuomilehto J, Lindstrom J, Eriksson JG, Valle TT, Hamalainen H, Ilanne-Parikka P, et al. Prevention of type 2 diabetes mellitus by changes in lifestyle among subjects with impaired glucose tolerance. *N Engl J Med* 2001;344(18):1343–50.

11. Data are taken from "The Human Genome Project": a CD produced and distributed by the National Human Genome Research Institute, National Institutes of Health. For information visit www.nhgri.nih.gov/educationkit.

12. ELSI looks at the following types of issues: interpretation of genetic knowledge; access to genetic data by law enforcement; the duty to warn; genetic profiling and discrimination in insurance or employment; and nature versus nurture in relation to the criminal justice system.

Index

obesity with hypo-ventilation 57–58

obstetrical experiences 15–19
  Caesarean section 35–36

Olivieri, Dr. Nancy 138

organs and tissues, "redundant" 239

organs and tissues, "renewable" 239

Ottawa Congress (1989) 237

ownership, organs and tissues 232

Oxford University xvii, 3, 253, 271
  St John Baptist College 4

"patient," an unsuitable word? 188

penicillin 4–6, 12–13, 20, 35, 152, 216, 218, 272
  bacterial endocarditis 12, 21, 218

pharmacy industry 136–39
  research funding 136, 138

physician incompetence 36, 38, 60–62

physician influence on patient decision 103

physician role in clinical research
  conflicts of interest:
    patient as research subject 216–18
    physician-investigator role 217

primum non nocere 33–36, 55

Quality of Life Committee (1984) 166–69, 171

Radcliffe-Richards, Prof. Janet 239

Rajotte, Dr. Ray 130–31, 142,

relational ethics 156, 262, 266, 268

repugnance, nature of 243

research subject, personal experience of 64

resource allocation issue
  India 157–59
  organs and tissues 232

Rolleston, Dr. Francis 223

Rothwell, D.J. 44

Royal Post-Grad. Hosp.
  Hammersmith 41–47, 71, 99, 216, 218

Royal Victoria Hospital (RVH) xvii, 48–49, 51–57, 62–63, 67, 72, 78, 81, 83, 85, 89–90, 99, 102, 107, 110–11, 113, 219
  Chief medical resident 52–62

sabbatical in medical ethics 172–76

Saidman, Dr. Susan 142, 153, 155

Sarcoidosis 26

Schaeffer, Dr. Otto 115, 119, 121

Schweitzer, Dr. Albert 145, 159, 242

Scribner, Dr. Belding x, 75–78, 80, 191

Sherlock, Dame Sheila xiii, 41–45, 56

skin grafts in Inuit in Igloolik 120

Smith, Donna, R.N. 177, 179, 204

St. Bartholomew's Hospital (Bart's) 4, 12, 15–16, 18, 20–21, 25–26, 37, 47–48, 51, 56, 134, 142, 175

Starzl, Dr. Tom 93–94, 106

stem cells 106, 129, 189, 237
  adult 95, 154
  toti-potential 12, 250

Stiller, Dr. Calvin R. xiii, 127, 237

Storch, Janet, Ph.D., R.N. xiii, 177, 179, 182

Summerskill, Dr. Bill xiii, 41, 71